Mental Health and HIV Infection

Mental Health and HIV Infection: Psychological and Psychiatric Aspects

Edited by

José Catalán

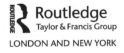

Routledge
Taylor & Francis Group

LONDON AND NEW YORK

First published 1999 in the UK and the USA
Reprinted 2003
By Routledge
11 New Fetter Lane, London EC4P 4EE

Transferred to Digital Printing 2003

The name of University College London (UCL) is a registered
trade mark used by UCL Press with the consent of the owner.

British Library Cataloguing in Publication Data
A catalogue record for this book is available from the British Library.

Library of Congress Cataloging in Publication Data
A catalogue record for this book has been requested

ISBN: 1-85728-170-5 HB
      1-85728-171-3 PB

Typeset by Best-set Ltd., Hong Kong

Social Aspects of AIDS

Series Editor: Peter Aggleton
(Institute of Education, University of London)

AIDS is not simply a concern for scientists, doctors and medical researchers, it has important social dimensions as well. These include individual, cultural and media responses to the epidemic, stigmatization and discrimination, counselling, care and health promotion. This series of books brings together work from many disciplines including psychology, sociology, cultural and media studies, anthropology, education and history. The titles will be of interest to the general reader, those involved in education and social research, and scientific researchers who want to examine the social aspects of AIDS.

Recent titles include:

Power and Community: Organizational and Cultural Responses to AIDS
Dennis Altman

Moral Threats and Dangerous Desires: AIDS in the News Media
Deborah Lupton

Last Served? Gendering the HIV Pandemic
Cindy Patton

Crossing Borders: Migration, Ethnicity and AIDS
Edited by Mary Haour-Knipe

Bisexualities and AIDS: International Perspectives
Edited by Peter Aggleton

Sexual Interactions and HIV Risk: New Conceptual Perspectives in European Research
Edited by Luc Van Campenhoudt, Mitchell Cohen, Gustavo Guizzardi and Dominique Hausser

AIDS: Activism and Alliances
Edited by Peter Aggleton, Peter Davies and Graham Hart

AIDS as a Gender Issue
Edited by Lorraine Sherr, Catherine Hankins and Lydia Bennett

Drug Injecting and HIV Infection: Global Dimensions and Local Responses
Edited by Gerry Stimson, Don C. Des Jarlais and Andrew Ball

Sexual Behaviour and HIV/AIDS in Europe: Comparisons of National Surveys
Edited by Michel Hubert, Nathalie Bajos and Theo Sandfort

Men Who Sell Sex: International Perspectives on Male Prostitution and AIDS
Edited by Peter Aggleton

The Dutch Response to HIV: Pragmatism and Consensus
Edited by Theo Sandfort

Social Aspects of AIDS
Series Editor: Peter Aggleton
Institute of Education, University of London

Editorial Advisory Board

Contents

Contents

Figures

Tables

Series Editor's Preface

An understanding of the mental health dimensions of HIV disease is vital to everyone involved in the care and support of people living with HIV and AIDS. Only by understanding the manner in which AIDS impact upon individuals, their friends, lovers and family can we plan the kinds of interventions that are required, and offer the understanding that is needed. In *Mental Health and HIV Infection*, José Catalán and contributors provide an overview of the major issues and problems that need to be addressed and the kinds of treatment and support that have proved most effective. As the long term prognosis for hundreds of thousands of people living with HIV disease improves, new challenges present themselves, not least those linked to the provision of medium to longer term therapy and care. A range of different therapeutic approaches is discussed and their strengths and weaknesses evaluated. Certain to become a standard reference text for health professionals and for informal sector carers, *Mental Health and HIV Infection* offers an overview of the key issues that need to be addressed and the most appropriate ways of providing care.

Peter Aggleton

Preface

It is now almost 20 years since the condition later known as AIDS was first identified, and much has been written about its medical, social and psychological consequences. This book attempts to review and discuss a range of topics related to the mental health impact of a disease that has affected many millions in developing and developed countries. Is there a need for a book on the psychological aspects of HIV? As a biased participant in the debate, I believe that it is relevant to focus on this particular dimension of HIV infection for several reasons: first, because the more severe psychological manifestations of the infection are often misunderstood by the general public, people with HIV and those involved in their care; second, as a mechanism to illustrate the range of effective ways of helping those experiencing mental difficulties in relation to HIV; and finally, as part of the process of examining the psychological and social consequences of the new antiretroviral treatments. Contrary to the mistaken belief held in some sectors that HIV has ceased to be a problem, it is essential to be reminded of the changing nature of the problems created by the infection – medical, social, psychological, economic – which will ensure we continue to face complex dilemmas for years to come.

Contributors to this volume have one thing in common: their direct and close involvement in providing care and support to people living with HIV and their families. It is from this hands-on personal commitment, often lasting many years, that their authority springs. In the case of Val, George and Adrian (Chapter 1), no further introduction is required. For the rest, their clinical and academic experience, listed at the end of the book, shows the extent and limits of their knowledge. I am grateful to them all for their responsiveness and efforts.

Gloria Davies provided much administrative help with a smile, and Kathryn Hill graciously allowed me the time to complete the task. Harry Dickinson, without realizing it, made the book possible. I am enormously grateful to them. Thanks are also due to Peter Aggleton who thought of this volume in the first place.

José Catalán

Chapter 1

Speaking in Tongues

Val, George and Adrian

I could think of no better way to illustrate the psychological consequences of HIV infection than to ask three people living with HIV to tell us how they have faced the persistent impact of their illness, treatment, and social reactions around them.

(the Editor)

Val: Talking of Labels

I am a 26-year-old HIV positive woman who 'suffers' from episodic 'schizophrenia'. I was an IDU (injecting drug user) for many years who also collected hepatitis C and B along the way. Given my own particular mental health problems, 90 per cent of my energy is diverted in maintaining mental stability. For when that goes, my life loses its perspective and form and I catapult toward a precipice of mental and physical decline. My equation works that way round, which says something about how psychosomatic HIV disease can be. The threat to life becomes a double bind: suicide from psychosis and death from opportunistic infection. But of course, it's not as cataclysmic as this all the time.

Being diagnosed HIV positive at the age of 15 was so singularly overwhelming that surviving AIDS became a project to attain a greater control over my life and to rid myself of the hype that AIDS equals death. If that sounds like I have the answer, I don't. But these are the psychological goals that seem to have enabled me to be here now, writing this, ten years after diagnosis. Or maybe they are simply the factors that I have most struggled with in the social and physical nightmare that HIV infection can bring. The basic answer to why have I survived this long is: I don't know. Maybe because I'm young, because I'm female, because my body was not in a state of worn disrepair at the time of infection; maybe I've had more tolerable infections than some others; maybe I've had more love and support. Probably I am just lucky.

To start at that place called *the beginning*, I suppose the first mental health aspect of HIV infection was being tested without my knowledge, let alone consent or counselling. Would I have got tested? By now, probably

1

yes, given the extent of symptoms. Back then, no. The idea would not even have occurred to me. Then young and healthy, my energies were deployed in a life of chaotic drug use; unable to cope with the chaos in my head, I discovered that heroin could very effectively – and pleasurably – stop my 'thinking'.

HIV diagnoses signalled the end of an era for many IDUs; time to get out and clean up. Never knowing th(os)e (romantic) 'carefree days of sex and drugs' before AIDS, I resented being too young and set apart from a chapter shared among many people I was now meeting. Yet my numbers had come up on the AIDS lottery, suddenly curtailing my own heroin project before it had really begun. I felt devastated about the infection and cheated out of my new lifestyle, mostly for the mental anguish that junk assuaged. Suddenly life seemed horribly serious.

The sensations of powerlessness that I have struggled against derive from having had negative labels appended to my person: being a minor; in *care*; under the jurisdiction of the courts and locked up as 'disturbed and out-of-control'; a drug addict with mental health problems, variously labelled from psychotic depression to schizophrenia and, of course, HIV positive. Despite the fact that *I* am lots (and lots) of other things as well, these merited no place at the category factory.

Negative labels are potentially disabling, because they locate and fix you within a specified agenda of 'this is what it is to be this'. I find it deeply patronising that people should be surprised that I have achieved what I have in my life; that I continued studying while shooting heroin (because I'm equally passionate about both), that I financed my drug habit through free-lance graphic design (because I find visual design problems stimulating) and that I went to university and came away with a starred first – after all, it's not what HIV+ schizophrenic IDUs do is it? Or is it? 'Chequered background' was the title awarded by my college at Oxford, making me a public curiosity of considerable social interest.

I was told by the hospital that I was not the only HIV positive under-graduate, but there was no way of meeting anyone else, and neither did it feel comfortable to; it felt far safer to keep these two worlds apart.

I found a simple act of faith in myself (what is needed most to fight this virus) very difficult to engender under these circumstances; until one day I considered biding Ibsen's advice: never commit the error of self-doubt. Ultimately, I *must* believe myself to be much more than the sum of the labels I am given. Fundamentally, this means defining where *I* stand in relation to the threat of AIDS.

Somebody recently described my outlook as 'positive denial'. Intellectu-ally I believe that HIV will kill me but in another sense I cannot believe it, and that's what keeps me going. I'm not looking for hard facts or concrete evi-dence, because there is none. If I did set out some kind of time plan or self-prognosis, it would render my life (i.e. merely the intervening period in the run-up to death) entirely meaningless.

I live completely for the work that I do, and the stimulation I derive from it. This I thrive on; certainly the strongest antiviral I ever got my hands on. I therefore take every recovery, whether from encephalitis or flu, as a personal triumph, a fact of my survival. My life from day to day, month to month, is about proving to myself that I am surviving.

By extension I have, sometimes ruthlessly, needed to eliminate those people and friends in my life who have accepted as a given that I will one day die of AIDS. Sadly, this also included my ex-partner, who was for many years the person involved with me most closely; who was the one to change the sheets in the middle of the night when I was shitting or vomiting in the bed, and who would be the one washing them the next morning while I slept in after my rough night. She was the one who came to the hospital every day, twice a day, because the house felt empty without me. And she was the one who saw me through my weakest moments of desperation, screaming and crying because I felt I just could not live like this anymore. These are the day-in day-out trials of living with HIV, the sum of which in many ways is a harder matrix to endure, because it can be relentless – the stream of niggling AIDS-ish symptoms with no specific drug therapy to blast them out.

But what I hung onto as an interlude – albeit an 18-month period of continuous illness and hospitalisation – she evidently could no longer see the end of, other than approaching the slope of perpetual decline. Maybe I under-estimated the sadness, terror and inevitable feeling of hopeless impotence that *she* faced. The other side of this is that my closest non-positive friends say I exude a something that lets them believe that somehow I will be okay. Whether I finally succumb or not becomes irrelevant. And if a prognosis really were anything to go by, I should certainly have died by now.

Succumbing to labels would also be to accept the widespread assumption that mental illness means you are a weak person, not simply that you face some kind of psychological vulnerability, and certainly not that you may yet function as a 'normal' individual in society, and achieve 'normal' goals. Admit-tedly, some people with enduring mental problems don't, but then some people severely ill with AIDS don't either. What is important is that there are many people, in both categories, who do. I am just one of them, and continue trying to be one of them.

Over a recent mental health crisis, a doctor friend managed to palliate my frustration and rage at being branded dysfunctional and irrational, when he explained that doctors were quite likely daunted by the 'complex medicine around me', saying that I warranted the three most stigmatized tags going: AIDS, IDU and mental illness. It seemed incredible – and ridiculous – that anybody should be *scared* by anything about *me*. I then thought about the vast disparity between me, myself and me, a set of loaded labels. That medicine works in response to these diagnostic and prognostic tags, and not to me, is epitomized by the zoning of my treatment; having to run between three clinics at three London hospitals (funding and contracts, you see), getting these various 'bits of me' seen to.

In many ways my mental health diagnosis has been the more isolating and harder to deal with. Partly, because a perspective on one's own psyche is difficult to form, especially if it periodically implodes. But principally, because there is no empowered 'community', waiting with outstretched arms to catch any stumbling members, as there was for HIV even in 1987, not to mention the vast support network there is now. But also, because people within the AIDS community share many of the misunderstandings and prejudices about mental health that exist in the whole population. As a result, this crucial part of myself – and in many ways for which I need the most support – has been boxed off in a separate and silenced compartment, the lid only forcing itself off at times of crisis.

In an act of self-protection, this made me even more withdrawn than mental illness already does. Heroin for me was a form of withdrawal, and administering it by needle an exercise of control over my body. Withdrawal also came through stopping speaking after being locked up when I was 15; and again, stopping eating the day a psychiatric nurse marched into my room with a pile of plastic plates and forks to enforce infection control. But ultimately, I was the one losing out each time.

The story of acting rather than reacting has been a recent phenomenon and one that was precipitated, ironically, by my first schizophrenic illness. I learn something more about myself every time I have to pick up the pieces and remake my personality.

Only very recently have I begun to be able to bridge these worlds through finding two people who are involved both with HIV and who work in mental health, and with whom I feel brave and safe enough to have made friends. Sharing this side of me has been an incredible release. Yet it is not just their special knowledge of both HIV and mental health, but the fact that they are good people; and I cannot stress enough the role that friends (both positive and not) have had in continuing to pull me through.

Just as my life hasn't rolled out according to its labelled agenda, so AIDS doesn't progress by any set pattern. It's different for everybody, and for any HIV positive individual things can also change all the time. On a practical level, surviving opportunistic infection is about prophylaxis, early intervention or effective management; dealing with symptoms early and fast is imperative.

There are many HIV positive people who have remained well for ten years or longer. Unfortunately, I started to become ill very shortly after diagnosis. I realise now that much of that early illness was due to my chaotic drug-using lifestyle. Cellulitis, abscesses, scepticaemia, endocarditis, the pleurisy and pneumonia of the heroin addict's depressed airways, all these are commonplace for the average junkie delivering substandard opiates directly into femoral veins. I realised that my junk sickness was fast moving in danger of becoming AIDS-defining illness, and decided now my turn had come to get out and clean up. But I was a little too late, for in the process of cleaning up I was diagnosed with tuberculosis (TB). But this only served to reinforce my project. Suddenly I felt urgency, mortality and an ardent desire to live, and live fully.

Most teenagers feel immortal, and I was no exception. Accepting my mortality took some believing and the risks that precipitated the early infections were like me testing my resilience. The stakes are lower now; dangerous games are no longer a way of life. Yet wild nights out are still there, and important. For there are no absolute concessions to be made to this virus. I have learnt to incorporate *it* into *my* life, and not the other way round. Hopefully I stay a few steps ahead of it, and keep moving forward.

I am holding off the new wonder stuff of combination therapy. My viral load came back last week at 130,000 particles per millilitre of blood. That's just into the margin of what is considered high, and I know of some who have had 800,000 particles reported. The upshot was an offer of triple combination therapy. Given the astronomical numbers of some, I returned from the clinic feeling rather pleased with mine, yet confused and somewhat bullied by the doctor who took my refusal of treatment as imprudent. Feeling overwhelmed by the range of new drugs and undecided over how much hope or certainty I could take from their astounding success in emptying AIDS wards, I phoned into the Terence Higgins Trust for advice, hoping that I would come away able to make an informed choice. But the counsellor's response replicated my doctor's and I put down the phone feeling faintly ridiculous for not running to the clinic with outstretched arms to embrace the pills that were going to save my life.

My resistance stems in part from a disastrous encounter with an alpha-interferon drug trial, which nearly killed me and whose chemotherapeutic effect so depressed my immune system after only a few weeks' injections that I spent all of 1995 in and out of hospital with infection after infection which culminated in a relapse of TB, but this time disseminated throughout my body. Of course the trial doctors will not to this day acknowledge any causal link, despite the fact that my CD4 count fell from 400 to 4 over the course of the interferon treatment (CD4 cells are a type of lymphocyte; they are also called helper T cells). Worse was the fact that I was not informed that this drug (apparently like any chemotherapy) had a very major side effect in depression. Knowing my mental health history, it felt tantamount to negligence that I was given this without being informed of the consequences, let alone being given any prophylactic antidepressants. Prior to going on the trial I had bought wholesale the doctors' story that this was the wonder cure to my liver disease and that any side effects were negligible. Subsequently, when I became so ill, I felt as though I had failed in some way, that I was not strong enough in body and mind to withstand this drug. Despite my ill health I attempted to get back on the trial for many months, which of course the hospital, terrified by my adverse reaction, would not agree to. It was only after I recovered and went in search of information about interferon that I learnt it was (subsequent to my adverse reaction) not to be given to HIV positive individuals without backup antiviral therapy (AZT, etc.), that it was categorically not to be given to people with mental health problems, and that I had being given a dose sufficient to intoxicate a huge male elephant. I know of at least one other (HIV negative) person who began the trial just before me and who also became very ill. And we were by no means the only ones devastated by the vicissitudes of this therapy. It infuriates me that my life was endangered because they needed an HIV positive guinea pig, and that I was thereby enlisted through lack of information.

Admittedly, the combination therapy story is diffferent, as are the nature of the drugs themselves. But without specialist medical knowledge as to how these pills and potions work in one's body it is extremely difficult to make informed choices; the other side of this is to passively take the word of those who say they have that knowledge.

Of course there have been many life-saving drugs and many exceptional doctors. My experience of medical care has been mostly positive, except perhaps in the early days, but then everyone was learning. And not all side effects are unwelcome. I am lucky to have found an antipsychotic drug that works for me and grants me some stability on a low maintainance dose. Further, this neuroleptic that in healthier days made me balloon hideously beyond my normal body weight, later rescued me from the emaciation of interferon therapy and today keeps me comfortably heavy. Ultimately, I allow myself credit for keeping myself well largely through my own means, with the unending support of those who love me.

Lastly, I was reflecting tonight after my co-author left to go home following our weekly meet to discuss this writing – a bottle of wine and many hilarious anecdotes later – how amazing is our capacity to enjoy ourselves, to laugh out loud, to make our lives good, full and enduring.

George: Living on Death Row

In 1980, aged 30, outwardly it seemed as if I really had it all going. I was the very model of a modern yuppie, or rather guppy, as I am a gay man. I had an extremely lucrative job as a copywriter in advertising and had already bought my bijou flat in Fulham. Yet inwardly I felt bereft, unfulfilled and unexplored. There was a void that needed exploring. I was just not happy with myself, particularly around my sexuality and gayness.

I felt I needed to celebrate and explore my gayness. To discover my otherness, my difference, and to feel proud of who I was. I needed to be rid of the piles of prejudice, ignorance and discrimination that I felt homosexual people have had heaped on them individually and collectively for far too long. This was the era of the gay community in San Francisco taking over the city and formulating an alternative, new sense of community where we, the traditional minority, could for once be the majority. A community with a fully formed network of political, business and social support systems. This was empowerment, and we gaily danced to the beat and rhythms of our own drums. Here one could be tender in public, and walk hand-in-hand without the fear of queer-bashing. Here gay people could start shedding the accumulated shame and guilt that blighted so many of us. Here was sexual politics in action. Here one had lots of sex with loads of men. These were the heady halcyon days of the Castro, *Tales of the City*, Harvey Milk. And here was just where I wanted to be.

Along with many other gay men from around the world, I decided to take the risk, sold my flat, and followed my Yellow Brick Road to the gay mecca of San Francisco. With appropriate gay abandon and gusto, for the next two years I threw myself, body and spirit, into this glorious challenge, and started to explore and fill the void. Life was a potent mix of sex and politics. These were the days just prior to the eruption of HIV into the world's consciousness. To us safer sex was an anathema, condoms a sign of repression, and a symbol of all we were trying to be rid of. Condoms had no place in our repertoire: they belonged elsewhere. And so we headed for the sex palaces to pleasure each other.

But in the fleshy backrooms and the steamy bathhouses we were tragically and unwittingly infecting each other with HIV, a disease that meant nothing could or would ever be the same again. The party was cruelly, sadly over. We had to adapt to survive and build new community solutions to support those of us living and dying with HIV.

I was recently trying to remember just what was my first realization of the hideous horrors that were just around the corner. My mind's eye goes back to Castro Street in 1982. I am strolling, on the way to brunch with my latest beau. We stop at the pharmacy window, and taped at the top of the glass window is a Polaroid close-up of a man's upper arm. Under the photo was a request for any gay man with such a lesion to go to the local sexual health clinic. The lesion was Kaposi's sarcoma, one of the first opportunistic infections. This one image, still vividly etched in my mind, heralded the onslaught of our very own holocaust. At that moment, I knew what the Jews of 1930s Europe must have felt when they first saw the swastikas of the Nazis.

And so slowly at first, then with alarming speed we began to succumb, sicken and die. I returned to England in late 1982. But I could not settle and readjust back into eighties England. I still felt an inner void. Another quest was called for; this time I wanted to immerse myself in the Oriental/Asian perspective. I took a job as a creative director for a big advertising agency in Bangkok. I soon met and fell wondrously in love with my Thai partner Sam, and we set to building a comfortable nest, and settled down to domestic bliss.

In 1985 on a holiday in the UK we both tested positive for HIV. We were not surprised, since with my sexual history they did not come much 'higher risk' than me. We carried on in Thailand until 1989. That year I developed an HIV-related cancer: a non-Hodgkin's lymphoma. I immediately returned to London for aggressive chemotherapy treatment. Sam followed six months later. This was the start of our dark and often terrifying days of life on the very front line of the pandemic.

This infection was certainly not the best thing to happen in my life, but was surely one of the most profoundly powerful and challenging experiences of my life. It was a personal earthquake that went to my very core, shattering all previous ambitions and life expectations. HIV has set me on a radically different and unexpected life path. Learning to coexist in some kind of harmony with this vile and vicious virus becomes a daily struggle against fierce and fearsome odds. As a result, many dark days began to plague me as I struggled to create my own unique coping strategies for survival. What follows are just a few of the feelings that these dark days throw up for me.

The Death Row Days are the fiercest. On these days I feel imprisoned and set in concrete by the fears and uncertainties that my HIV status presents. These fears are my cell, guard and locks. As I wait on Death Row, I see my cellmates, friends and even partner, one by one shrink and shrivel away before me in cruel and undignified deaths, and I howl at the Moon in rage at the sheer waste and hopelessness of it all. On such days I feel I am reduced to nothing more than tea and sympathy, yet with blessings, somehow I live as all around me die. Then there are the Abyss Days, days when it seems the losses will never end, and the cumulative effect of constant loss pushes me to the very edge of the abyss.

But yet I stand back, observe, and live on

The Panic Days are dire indeed. Days when a bruise is Kaposi's sarcoma, a cough is PCP (pneumocystic pneumonia), a bump becomes a tumour, and a headache becomes toxoplasmosis. The list of potentially life-threatening opportunistic infections waiting to pounce and carry me away seems awesome and mammoth. It feels as though I am living an abbreviated life, a life poised on a knife-edge of fear. At such times being positive seems nothing more than an empty, trite cliché. The No Days are, for me, a common occurrence; moments when there appears to be absolutely no hope, no help, no future, no energy, no choices and no cure. Then I feel hopeless and helpless, alone and lonely, unloved and unloveable.

But still I cope; still I go on

The Feeling-Old Days are stressful times when I feel robbed of my potential, my future and the choices other people take for granted. I feel as if I have been catapulted into old age without a middle age in which to prepare. Here all is clinics and crematoria, death and dying. Yet I struggle on in my own way.

The Alien Days are complex. I feel I am a twentieth-century leper, diseased, different and discriminated against. The sting of social shame and stigma from the ignorant and fearful lashes deep into my self-esteem. I see the rejection and pity in others' eyes and hear the wicked spouting of the judgemental moralists, 'Serves them right, it's an own goal,' and I wish the Dalai Lama was Pope. Such utterings make me despair and question just how civilized a society we live in. As a gay man, I am well used to such alienation and living proudly and openly with HIV has been a difficult coming out for me.

But I try to move on

Survivor guilt is, for me, extremely difficult to deal with. These are my Why Not Me Days. Why my partner Sam, why Carl, Antoinette, Bill, Rod, Steve, David . . . ? Why friends and friends of friends and always it comes back to why not me? And then, when me? It feels like I am in another Holocaust. At such moments I feel powerless. It is as if I am just waiting my turn, hosting a time bomb waiting to explode. But, so far, it hasn't.

And I live on

The Angry Days hit often and are sparked off by a variety of means. They bubble up inside and cascade out. I do feel angry and let down by the medical and scientific professions. After 15 years and their combined might, there is still no cure. The virus still outfoxes them. I am angry at the drug companies and their profiteering attitude and provision of exorbitantly priced drug therapies. It feels as if they grow fat on our suffering. The quacks, charlatans and tricksters who have peddled false hope through pills, potions and cures are despicable and one gets easily angry with them. The shocking initial neglect and lack of real practical support by the likes of Reagan and Thatcher was outrageous and typical. We were 'not one of us'. We were 'one of them' incarnate, and suffered accordingly. This angers me.

The careerists and growing AIDS establishments born of the pandemic, who can often be self-seekers promoting their own agenda rather than ours, seem as if they too have clambered on board our wagon of trouble. Many are second-rate and provide second-rate, costly services. When I try to think just how it must be like to be living with HIV/AIDS in the developing countries of Africa, Asia and South America, I despair. I feel anger at the lack of choices and treatments that they can access. At best, they are guinea pigs for the drugs barons on which they can test their latest concoctions. I take for granted so much of the HIV network of support available to me.

I also rage when I hear people saying that because of combination therapy, people are cured. People are no longer infectious. People can practise unsafe sex. And I anger that after all the years of education and our examples, people are still getting infected. I dislike the continual assessing, processing, reviewing and interview processes that it feels I continually have to undergo. It feels demoralizing to have to open up to clipboard-carrying strangers of whom you know nothing. I end up feeling like a raw statistic to be fed into the inevitable computer.

I get very angry when I remember the cruel way the Immigration Office and Home Office treated Sam and me. Sam gave up his job, family, country and culture to care for me in 1989. When we applied for permission for him to stay as my carer and work, some official wrote back saying he could not work because our relationship was not 'normal', was not 'acceptable'. It broke my heart and Sam's spirit.

I find negotiating safer sex very difficult. It is sad when I am rejected just because I am positive. I do not wish to lose my sexuality to the virus, but it is a struggle for me to find the pleasures and excitements of safer sex. I explore touch and intimacy much more recently. Often I feel boundaried to the point of patronization. I rile at the 'we know best' school of service care: rigid, inflexible, rule-book boundaries, and those that practise them have left me often feeling less connected, more isolated. Some days, sadly, I am still that little bit angry at Sam for dying and leaving me to die alone.

The Cotton Wool days can be demanding. I awake and it immediately feels as if the day is tainted; no longer neutral. It is as if the day has something threatening hanging over it. Something like an interview, an operation, an exam, a funeral. . . . When the virus drains you of every last drop of energy, particularly after exhausting night sweats, I feel very fragile, very weak. The smallest effort becomes gargantuan, and I feel sick and tired of being sick and tired, and wish no longer to go on merely coping, merely existing. At such moments I pull the bedcovers tightly over my head, and like a hermit crab withdraw inside my Teflon-covered isolation bubble. And I wait for the energy to come back.

The Living Dead or Lazarus Days are a fairly recent message of the pandemic. For over nine years I was told I was facing an imminent death. I have, accordingly, been busy adjusting my life and attitudes for such a death. Now someone has come knocking on my coffin lid announcing that I got it hideously wrong. I am not going to die, but live, especially if I take the tablets. Now the real pressure is to get up and get back to work as if everything is as it was before diagnosis. If people genuinely feel fully fit, able and willing to return to work, so be it. But to those of us who believe that surviving with HIV is one's life's work, then we should have the choice. It does not feel, to me, that the choice is available.

Yet, despite this list of dark and cheerless days, having the virus has shown me many wondrous, bright days of bliss and contentment. Days of real happiness and harmony. Days of going beyond loss into new opportunities that have allowed me to form a whole new philosophy and spirituality.

In order to change these dark days to bright, I have created and cobbled together my very own life raft in which I have blessedly managed to steer a safe course through the perils of stormy seas, and troubled times. This raft has successfully carried me through two bouts of HIV-related cancers and the subsequent treatments, the loss of Sam, my beloved partner of ten years, and has shone a light upon the dark days and feelings. I have built my life raft out of the wreckage of my pre-positive life, shedding great chunks of what was no longer necessary or valid, while I sifted my way through the mountain of information, people and systems that diagnosis presents. A daunting and demanding task. What follows now are some of the planks and parts of my life raft; some of my coping strategies that may hold clues as to why I still live on.

Upon my diagnosis (D-Day I call it), I realised that it was to be the first day of the rest of my life. The first thing I decided to do was to allow myself truly to open up to the virus, and start preparing myself in body, mind and spirit for the inevitable struggles, challenges and losses that would follow. I could no longer rely on my pre-diagnosis coping strategies. Things would never be the same. I quickly accepted that from now on HIV was as much a part of my body as my brain. It was a physical part of me – a medical fact.

I had to learn about the virus and I began sifting through information that I felt would empower and strengthen me in the battles ahead. I also released myself from any personal and projected feelings of guilt or shame about being positive. It was a fact; no more, no less. I soon realised that the best I could realistically hope to achieve was to learn to coexist in harmony with the virus. I had to keep it dormant, and stop it activating at all costs.

I need to try and find out for myself ways of going beyond the fears, beyond the losses and find new beginnings. I began crafting a personal philosophy around this, a philosophy that has in many ways been the missing piece in my own jigsaw puzzle. I felt that a life lived in constant fear of the virus was a quick way to activate it. I also acknowledged that I was facing a real and possible threat of imminent death. I had not previously prepared or faced up to this issue, so I began a deep inner search for the peace and strength to deal with this huge issue.

I began truly to seize the moment. I saw that the time left to me was very special, almost sacred. I wanted, in my own way, to relish and savour every last moment of it. It was clear that from now on my very concept of time and future had to change. No longer the grandiose goals and long-term ambitions. Just the simple joys of the everyday, the here and now.

In my pre-positive life, my frantic and frenetic quest for fame, fortune and goodies took its toll on me. To survive this part of my life I had to be highly competitive and ambitious. I was not that pleasant to be around; I was hard. In this process I had badly neglected the appreciation and nurturing of my spiritual and emotional needs. I felt unfocused, immature and underdeveloped. I was asleep. In California I became interested in Zen Buddhism, and unearthed a simple way to wake myself up from my spiritual slumber.

It was the simple yet magical words and wisdom of the Buddha's teachings that lit me up and turned me inwards on a journey to untangle and unearth my own path. My ten years of living and working in Asia, and my relationship with Sam deepened my understanding and practice of life lived in the Middle Way – the Buddhist way. I had long ago dismissed the external god-figure philosophies of orthodox religions. For me, god is within, so it is within I have gone to directly access the powers of my own god-force. To connect with this often neglected yet powerful source, the teachings of Buddha opened up an entrance and a path out of my often deep personal darkness. It offered me light again.

Through meditation I try to keep myself in balance, harmony and equilibrium. By stilling my mind I can still the fears. My belief in reincarnation has lessened the fear of death, yet still the process of dying terrifies me. It has encouraged me to be kinder and more mindful of both myself and others, and has knocked off many of my harder edges. It has allowed me actually to start getting to know myself and even like myself. It encourages me to respect mind, body and spirit if I wish to stay in harmony and balance. I also love the pagan and animistic powers of nature and magic, and I am a natural tree and stone hugger. My personal spiritual, inner beliefs are a major plank in my life raft. They give me great succour and strength. Indeed, it is probably the very sail under which I sail down the tricky path fate has ordained for me.

And so I sail on

In place of the initial fear and terror, I began in a strange way to respect the virus. For 15 years this clever little bug has managed to keep one vital step ahead of the combined might of the world's boffins. I started to cherish and nurture myself; commonsense stuff, really. I learned to read my body; I discovered the power of fresh foods, a nutritious diet and the creative pleasures of cooking – things I had previously neglected. I shed a great deal of accumulated excess baggage in the form of people and inappropriate attitudes. I reached out to the power, love and support of a small group of true friends who still gently keep a caring eye on me. The love of Sam, my beloved partner who died of AIDS three years ago, was wonderfully strengthening and soothing; I miss it, and him, dreadfully.

One of the most exciting ideas to come out of the epidemic was the formulation of a completely new holistic model of health and patient care. Medical practice shifted away from the traditional, paternalistic 'doctor knows best' attitude, and moved towards encouraging patients' autonomy with greater involvement and information sharing in making joint decisions about treatment options. Medical decisions now considered the specific needs of the whole individual. And the best way to establish them is simple: ask the patient, listen and provide time and space for discussion. This positive partnership model offered a whole lot more than 'the tablets' for the whole of the person.

In the early years of the pandemic, this model was picked up and applied by various service provider professionals (nursing, social work, GPs, psychiatry). It provided some inspiring pioneer work and people. Sadly, it feels as if this founding passion is largely gone today. An almost historical and old-fashioned idea. I regret this very much and feel we need to rediscover this alternative model of health care, one that can be a useful role model across the NHS for all groups of people struggling with life-threatening illnesses. I gathered around me a support team to cover all of my holistic treatment needs, all of them dedicated to the holistic approach of patient care. Their input is simply huge, and I have great respect for the way they have skilfully helped me steer myself through many medical challenges. I also like them as individuals, and see them in many ways as a special set of friends. I hope we are not currently seriously in danger of losing all the invaluable work done up to now, by many people in a variety of areas.

I stopped full-time work in 1989 when my first HIV cancer struck. I felt that as I had already had a successful and fulfilling career, stopping work was not for me the loss that it is for many positive people. Surviving and thriving became my new life's work. The pay is bad, but it provides more challenges than working in an office. I relished the idea of having this extra free time, and began to develop interests that I had thought would have to wait until retirement and old age. I discovered the sheer joy of gardening and began to create collages from discarded and found objects.

For me, these interests became effective ways to restore my sometimes shaky feelings of self-worth. They increased my sense of achievement and raised my flagging and battered self-esteem. I recognized my need to be involved with the wider positive community and felt a need to give back and share my experiences. I started with media work, speaking publicly and putting a face to the statistics of the pandemic. I have also visited schools and answered questions, particularly around safer-sex messages. This has, in turn, enabled me to feel connected, to feel valid, less isolated.

I quickly tapped in to the wonderfully restorative powers that are offered by complementary therapies, my two personal favourites being aromatherapy and acupuncture. Although many people living with HIV have seemingly benefited from combination therapy, I am still treatment-naive. I am blessed with a naturally low viral load, a good immune system, and a reasonable CD4 count. I believe my long-term use of marijuana has been effective in handling stress, sleep, appetite and pain control. I am a firm advocate of the legalization of medicinal marijuana. I do not, and have never taken, chemical recreational drugs.

My flat has become very special for me as I spend so much time there. Here I can truly feel safe and distanced from the harsh and sometimes cruel realities of the world outside my door. On bleak, despondent days I often open my personal memory box of magic moments. I dip in and select a memory and carefully try to capture and savour the beauty of that time. From a rainy, lonely London day I can be making love in a beach hut in Bali; sitting atop a pagoda in Burma; or even riding an elephant in the Thai rainforest, picking wild orchids. I live alone now, quite contentedly if somewhat passionlessly. I do miss not being in love. Perhaps for the first time ever, I now live by, for and with myself, and I can truly live life just how I want to with exactly whom I like.

The virus has systematically stripped away so much of my pre-positive lifestyle with its demanding responsibilities and commitments. With those largely gone, life has never been simpler. I have worked long and hard at getting to know myself and generally am quite fond of who I am, so living with myself is not problematic. I have spent many hours in my own mental and spiritual gym. I do not fear solitude; in fact, I relish it. Stillness and silence are very valuable to me. So I have no fear of living on my own, and indeed enjoy it.

I do not offer my life raft as any instant panacea for survival or as a quick guide to building effective coping strategies. This is just how it is, and how it feels for me. This is how I approach it. These are just a few of the composite parts of my raft, one that is unique to me and formed out of who and what I am. Namely a White, gay, middle-aged man. Just how each of us deals with the task of building our very own rafts is, for me, one of the great wonders of life. Observing how we construct our lives, some of us never even start, others start too late, others choose inappropriate materials, and many seem unable to put it all together. Many sink at the first ripple, others spring leaks and go under. Many are smashed to bits by the pounding waves, and yet others run aground on hidden menaces. And many just seem unable to steer or navigate their rafts and end up hopelessly lost.

Mine is definitely the worse for wear. The sail is battered and torn, the hull has sprung many a leak, but it still holds fast. I am sure there are still troubled seas and battering storms ahead, but then I have never wanted a life lived in the doldrums.

And so, on I sail, and with blessings, I still live on, on Death Row

Adrian: A Story of Doctor and Patient

What difficulties have you faced and how have you overcome them to survive AIDS for so long? That's the question, and already I'm uneasy. If I have overcome, conquered and triumphed, did my dead friends, and dead friends of friends fail? No, they died difficult deaths, having lived with long illnesses. They all went over the wire, didn't they? They didn't fail.

If asked why I think I've lived longer than many, at the bottom of it, I think it's the genes – my genes and the viral genes. My immunity's held up for a bit longer because my viruses can only destroy my immune system slower than other varieties of the virus can destroy others' immune systems. It can be so fast. For instance, Jack died a hard death within 18 months of infection. It's a bell curve of survival, some quick, some slow, and I happen to be well over on one side.

The AIDS decline, like the cancer decline, is classic horror – wasting, disfigurement, pain, dementia and dependence, soiled beds and skin all sores. Slow or fast, the decline has seemed almost inevitable. Bodies weakened by the virus and then overwhelmed by bugs from the dung of cattle, pigeons and cats, bugs that have been here for years, held dormant by the immune system that has now collapsed. If not these, then one of more than a hundred other opportunistic options on the menu.

I've had AIDS for seven years (by United States diagnostic rules), and five years (by United Kingdom rules). I may or may not officially be a long-term survivor – the rules for that are mysteriously changed too. It used to be five years after a diagnosis, but it's often restricted to those diagnosed before 1988. Or maybe it's ten years after diagnosis. Either way, they are the old crowd, the HIV industry.

I've been on bug poison since this all started for me, one April morning in 1990, and as if jumping from piece of driftwood to piece of driftwood after a shipwreck, new drugs have become available just as I needed them, as my health started to fade on the last new drug.

I started AZT (azidothymidine) the day of my first and positive HIV test, as I had AIDS-related symptoms. My first CD4 count the next week was 30, critically low and usually terminal. The drug poisoned me more than the bug, and I needed eight pints of blood after just eight weeks of treatment. I was lucky. DDI (dideoxyinosine) was just available, fresh from a test tube, and I took it for three years successfully, until that started to fail. My day-to-day symptoms – the symptoms of AIDS, rather than of an opportunistic infection or cancer – were a burden again late in 1993. D4T (stavudine) just arrived in time, and I was reprieved again for three years or so.

By the winter of 1995–6 I was fading again fast. That winter of 1995–6 I had ten chest infections, lost weight I couldn't put back and shat fluid ten times a day. With AIDS one's whole body is sick – aches and pains, skin rashes, guts, hair loss, and so on. Self-esteem and confidence take a bashing as you slim.

The new wonder drugs came to the UK in December 1995, and I was one of the first people in the UK to start them, in January 1996. That began what proved to be both my toughest and yet my most optimistic year. In the spring, after three months of combination therapy, I still wasn't well. My guts worsened during the year despite the promise. My body wasn't absorbing vitamins or medication properly. I was wasting.

In June I was working in Dublin, and had trouble brushing my teeth one morning. I'm a doctor, and I knew this was a brain problem, but as always in the first few days of an opportunistic infection, I just denied it to myself. There's always a delay before I seek help. This is a dangerous denial, quite different from the other denial. Although I accept I am in a serious situation, I deny I will die from it. I am someone who might be termed a *positive denier*, a term from studies of women with breast cancer. There's a rumour from the research that we survive best of all. Back in London the next week and unable to write on students' papers, I couldn't deny any longer and rang my doctor.

I've seen the same doctor almost since the beginning. He, the nurses, the specialist clinical staff and all the other people who work there are among the keys to my survival. They are excellent. I am also lucky that when the axe fell, wealthy friends found me a place to live near the clinic. That accessibility has been crucial during health crises.

Not all health workers are like these people. I never realised why patients so often complain about health workers, and especially doctors. You see I'm a gamekeeper turned poacher; to quote some of today's newspaper headlines, I'm one of the HIV doctors. And now I'm a patient too, I understand. I have been treated appallingly throughout the system on some occasions, as well as very well on others. Bullying and rude staff are common, and are just generally offensive to everyone. Waiting three hours, and never being told when anything's going to happen, is not uncommon. Being treated as stupid is endemic in the system.

I had thought when people complained about doctors, why? We all work hard, study hard, know so much about your disease. Haven't we made you better? But that general knowledge of a disease doesn't tell us what that disease, and its treatment, is like in someone's life. But we presume we know what to do. We do not advise, we often order stupidly, and when the treatments fail, we blame the patient.

My worst experience was with surgeons. Having anal warts and AIDS upset the homophobic surgeons, and on both occasions the treatment was appalling. The rudeness, the barely concealed contempt, the repeated cancellation of my operation because I was a 'dirty case', and the unethical premedication for an operation, followed by its cancellation – Oh, sleep it off and go home. I had to fight to get pain relief after their sick medieval practice – the burning up and scarring of gay arseholes with red-hot rods, masquerading as surgery. Remember how they killed Edward II. You don't need to be a psychoanalyst to see the hatred and perversion in this treatment that leaves every shit an agony for a month and doesn't work – the warts just come back. When finally I was told 'bugger's bums' are offensive to treat, I complained. The professor of surgery sneered, and the director of the HIV clinic loftily declared no discrimination had taken place. I lost a lot of confidence in the system. I learnt never complain to doctors about doctors, but to go to managers and chief executives. What finally worked was my tantrums, my good doctor and my knowledge of the system, and a good and kind surgeon in a good and kind dedicated hospital 'for diseases of the anus and rectum'. I am still angry five years later.

But back to June 1996, unable to write, I rang my good doctor, and my head was in a washing machine scanner within hours. An hour later he told me it was serious, the possibilities were grim, but for a better answer I was sent to an MRI scanner (magnetic resonance imaging) the next day. He also gave me his home phone number for my brother to ring, and in case I needed it – a kind gesture. The nurses in the clinic couldn't look at me as I left. I was scared.

The second scan was frightening. I had to lie down and my head was restrained with foam wedges and Velcro straps, preventing any movement. A row of metal bars was lowered over my face – jokes about the *Silence of the Lambs* are apparently common at this point. I had earplugs in to protect me against the noise of the machine, but also amplifying my isolation. I was then drawn into the long narrow tunnel of the machine, and the room emptied as the kind staff disappeared behind protective doors. Enclosed down to below my knees, I had a mirror to see out, but the claustrophobia was intense. It was like the coffin I had been told I would probably soon be in. I was practising to use a quadriplegia mirror, and to be buried alive at the same time. I was in there panicking for almost an hour. I was thinking, so this is how I ended, this is what got me in the end. I have known for seven years that this day could always be tomorrow, and now it was that long-dreaded tomorrow today. As I left I opened the MRI report – PML.

I had missed PML (progressive multifocal leukoencephalopathy) in the small print of AIDS up until now. The organization Gay Men's Health Crisis described it as 'probably the worst AIDS diagnosis'. While I don't want to have an argument about one AIDS diagnosis being worse than another, it was terrifying to have the purported worst manifestation of this, the worst of all illnesses, AIDS. This virus – the JC virus (as in: get to meet Jesus Christ virus) – would destroy the white matter of my brain over eight to twelve weeks, leaving me locked in, deaf, unable to move, speak, communicate with anyone I loved. No mention of dementia, no oblivion, no sweet release to look forward to. I would be conscious more or less to the end, which might be in September. My doctor promised he would care for me until then. I wanted to die now, today, with my own hand before I lost the power of it.

They took fluid off my brain from my spine a couple of days later, and the consequent headaches, incapacity and vomiting lasted for two of those eight weeks, two of my precious eight weeks. Pain like I had never known. This scared everyone who was caring for me because it seemed like I was already terminally ill. The painkillers they gave me made my ears ring, and I wept in my lover's arms, believing the bug had started on my ears already, and soon I would never hear music again.

Friends mobilized swiftly, and started arriving with flowers, shopping and cash. A group of maybe twenty people began to collect protectively around me, and I felt, amazingly in the circumstances, safe. I would not die alone. I think without these people – and many don't have these people in their lives – I would have died from the fear. The individual acts of kindness I will never forget. I will always think of the clinic and these friends if asked how I coped.

One friend went to Star Information Exchange for information, and found a PML survivors and carers group in Los Angeles. Within three days a chain of people (many of whom I'll never meet) found the group, and information was Fed Ex-ed from LA and biked to my door. Such communication the gay community is justly proud of. It seemed, in fact, not quite so fatal. Ten per cent of people got better, ten per cent got no worse. The agony of hope again after the despair.

I fled with my lover to a dear friend and his house in a wood by the sea in France to try to be one of those ten percents. I didn't deteriorate during the month in France. Nothing in my body changed. I swam, played tennis (after a fashion) and I sure could still talk. I came back to London, saw my good doctor and was sent back to the coffin for a third scan. Little panic this time. This scan showed that all I had was two or three mild strokes, which were much better now. I had to take a quarter aspirin a day for life, and everything would be fine. 'It's good news', my doctor said. 'It's not as simple as that', I replied. This had been a mock execution. The gun had been empty after all. It had been a cruel dress rehearsal for the people who love me? Will they or I ever be able to do it again if I'm here again?

I emerged into a very different world from the one I had left with the mock execution. Only six to seven weeks away from the world, preparing to die. Now I returned to an AIDS world where the news was that combination therapy was working. My own combination therapy had started to work about August, after six or seven months of treatment. I think this delay was because my guts were so bad at the beginning of the year, I absorbed very little to begin with. I was very ill and my system was very depleted – I was close to dying. My recovery from there has been very slow. Now, after a year on the tablets, I am well and almost completely free of the symptoms. My guts are good, I can eat what I want, and so on. No friend or friend of a friend has died for six months (though a couple are ill). People are gaining weight and energy, and talking about what now in their lives. I am stepping back on the medical career ladder. New dawn or false hope?

I expect the combination to work for three years or so, as the other drugs did for me and then I will fade again. If they do no more, the gain for me has been immense. A taste of health again; allowing myself to dream of life in two or three years' time, after so many years never believing I could live more than six months; that I am alive now at all. There is a price. I have to fast for three hours, three times a day, and take twenty-odd tablets five times a day. I think it's a better deal than for a diabetic. Not bad for the gain. Will it last? Will it have some scary sting in the tail – give us all leukaemia or liver cancer in two years' time?

I had always dreaded dying just when the cure came out. It was an old fantasy, since shortly after being diagnosed. This summer the nightmare happened to me – it seemed like I was going to be one of the last people to die of AIDS. Though I was reprieved, I feel very aware that the treatment does fail. There are others who don't respond, and moreover, it fails just about everybody with AIDS who lives outside Europe, and may yet fail me.

I haven't sought much mental health care. I was in therapy when I was diagnosed, but left shortly afterwards. My family failed to cope with my diagnosis, and that seemed too real for Jungery, and the mystery of the transference.

I feel spared a lot of therapy by fate. I had PCP, the AIDS fungal pneumonia, and was quite ill. This was my AIDS-defining event (UK rules), my first communion, so to speak. In the four weeks afterwards my father and I began to sort ourselves out. He hadn't spoken to me for the first two years after my diagnosis, after a lifetime of not speaking to me very much. We finally had lunch and we kissed goodbye for the first time in 25 years. He died, out of the blue, the next day, from a ruptured heart. My brother and I spoke for the first time since my diagnosis in the intensive care sitting room, in the hours my dad was dying on an operating table. The ravages of PCP had me looking like a corpse at his funeral. Whose funeral is this? Have they put the wrong person in the box? It was like being in a bad movie, but it was happening. However, I now think that if by chance things had been the other way around, if the PCP had followed my father's death, some therapist would have always had me believe my grief had led to my PCP. For many hundreds of hours of therapy.

I went to see a wonderful psychiatrist after the mock execution. I asked to go really to communicate to the good doctor how traumatic it had all been, and because I felt so unreal. The psychiatrist didn't pathologize me and offer therapy, rather he empowered me by asking me to write all this.

He asked me to think of what has been important. I don't think life events change the course so much. Big nights out take their toil. My AIDS symptoms used to flare up after a binge, but then settle again in a few days. I've kept up big nights out throughout, though there's some pressure to stop. Stress from toxins is one angle. According to this view, the AIDS body is dirty, and must be spared drugs and alcohol, meat and smoke, and be offered water, vegetables and rest. Some people party to the grave. Others seem scared and seem never to want to cope. Over several months they slowly fade, physically and spiritually, and finally float off in the early hours of one morning. I spent the first four years of AIDS giving up and restarting to smoke cigarettes. I quit three years ago, but smoked a fair bit of grass as a substitute for three years until I knocked it on the head. But big nights out, binges, partying in queer street is important to me. In that spiritual shanty town we've built out of the scraps left us by straight culture – and by we I don't mean just gay men and lesbians, but a host of people from other sexual minority groups, and a fair number of straight women who belong as much as anyone – I find things that are important to me.

I believe the echo between the secret of being gay and the secret of the infection, grotesque though it is, has given me skills at coping with stigma, with difference, and so on. What is it like never to have been persecuted, to be persecuted now? The solidarity of the queer community, though not perfect, I think has been a pillar.

Half of my positive friends are gay men, and half straight women, mainly drug-using women who got infected one way or another. There are of course conversations that one can only have with another positive person. Such is the way of these things. I fell out with one group of gay male positive friends though, because they were fiercely antimedication, and were dying, and were bullying other people off their drugs. As my health slipped, I just couldn't take their insistence my condition was a result of the antivirals, rather than the viruses. Fine, find your own way through AIDS, but don't ask me to follow you.

Some say the AIDS industry is now turning quite straight. The yuppies are again stepping into the shoes of dead men and women. I always found the industry people frightening, glamorous and confident, and I feel as if I'm not hip enough for the club. I do value two magazines, *Body Positive* and *Aids Treatment News*. It's sad that many people don't get them, because information is poor. It sometimes seems the attitude is: You're gay, you know what's what.

Stress from work is another. For me employment is important and relaxing; the boredom of unemployment, stressful. I have carried on working as a doctor with considerable support from a number of senior colleagues. These doctors and other professionals have been exceptional, and not only have I continued to work part-time, but I have a small area of expertise all of my own. I want to tell you about my work, but I fear being identified. One person has used the information about my health to undermine me at work, and she caused me a lot of stress. I even wonder if her barely concealed revulsion and subsequent bullying led to my strokes. I fortunately had enough power to ensure that I no longer work anywhere near her. Enough nastiness will make anyone ill, and there's plenty of research on that one. I curse her now.

I want you to know that though I was so ill, I continued to work, as others can and should. For many people work gives purpose, and it has kept me alive, I'm sure. But I fear the prejudice. Working part-time matters, and it matters to know why. The great mistake, when choosing to work part-time because you want more time for other things, is to believe it is because you are too ill to work. This simple mistake is a great disabler for people with AIDS. A good part-time job gives money, purpose and involvement, whereas staying at home on benefits can leave a person worried about poverty, bored and feeling pointless. My medical knowledge has helped more than I can say in enabling me to understand my predicament and my options. Information really is power.

If it is over, which I doubt, why did all those people, among them my friends, and that world, have to die? I have changed so much from all of this and like myself much more than before all of this. I thought during those years that to have AIDS and then survive, to learn so much about life from being so close, so very close to death through AIDS, and then to live, surely that would be a life lived with some enlightenment. Now, they hint, I may be one of the first to survive, but of course cruelly I may still be one of the last, or one of the many more to die.

Chapter 2

Psychological Problems in People with HIV Infection

José Catalán

This chapter reviews the profound psychological consequences which may result from HIV infection. It examines the psychological profile of individuals seeking HIV testing, the impact of notification of infection, and the problems of asymptomatic and symptomatic individuals. The introduction of new anti-HIV treatment in recent years has produced important changes in the pattern of psychological adjustment for people with HIV infection, and some of these new issues are discussed here.

Introduction

The adverse psychological and social consequences of HIV have been known since the start of the epidemic, and their recognition by people with HIV, their advocates and carers, has over the years contributed to shape the way public responses to the infection have been articulated. At the same time, the severity of the psychological distress and hopelessness experienced by people living with HIV could be seen as an indicator of how HIV/AIDS is socially perceived at a particular time and in a particular place.

As the second decade of the epidemic comes to a close, it is important to establish what we know about the psychological impact of HIV, and what new psychological issues arise as treatment strategies evolve and the clinical picture and prognosis of the infection change. There is at present a feeling that the textbooks will have to be rewritten soon and that what was thought to be certain knowledge will be shown to be less solid than expected. Developing hope seems easy at the moment, but sustaining it over the longer term may prove more difficult. It is early days and we have only limited evidence of what the impact of the new anti-HIV treatments is on the psychological status of people living with HIV, and no doubt new research will become available in the near future, mapping out what is expected to be a more optimistic picture of the way people with HIV cope with their predicament. It is important to remember, however, the continuation of unequal access to care accross the globe, and the differences not only between developing and developed countries, but within different socio-economic groups in developed countries.

HIV and Mental Health Problems

HIV infection has been associated with a broad range of mental health problems, including not only what could be regarded as understandable emotional reactions to a potentially fatal illness, with a substantial stigma attached to it, but also frank psychiatric disorders, such as major depression, and neuropsychiatric syndromes, such as HIV-associated dementia. Understandable emotional reactions, such as distress, shock, anger or regret, are extremely common and need not be considered abnormal unless they become very severe or persistent and substantially interfere with the person's life and social adjustment.

Psychiatric disorders are more likely to develop in vulnerable individuals as a result of the interaction between the person, the stressful situation and the social and emotional supports available. Neuropsychiatric syndromes are the result of the direct or indirect effects upon the brain of HIV or from complications resulting from the individual's immunosupression, such as opportunistic infections or tumours. This chapter gives an overview of the emotional reactions and psychiatric disorders that can develop at different stages of HIV infection. Related topics are covered elsewhere: suicidal behaviour in Chapter 6, euthanasia and doctor-assisted suicide in Chapter 7, and HIV-associated dementia in Chapter 5.

HIV and Development of Mental Disorders

In spite of the many health and social problems faced by people with HIV infection, it is a remarkable fact that many find effective ways of coping successfully with the impact of the infection, making use of personal and external resources to deal with the difficulties, and at the same time avoiding the development of mental health problems. A substantial proportion, however, experience important mental health difficulties, and it is important to identify the factors that make such problems likely, so as to prevent their onset if at all possible by modifying these causal factors, or else by means of early identification of people experiencing problems.

HIV-Related Factors

Mental health problems are more likely to occur at two stages: when the person is given a diagnosis of HIV infection, and when physical symptoms develop or worsen. The distress associated with notification of a positive HIV test result is usually self-limited, but the way the news is given, the individual's expectation of the result, disclosure to others, and the degree of support available will influence the course and duration of the difficulties (Ostrow *et al.*, 1989; Pergami *et al.*, 1994; Davis *et al.*, 1995; Holt *et al.*, 1998).

According to many studies, the development of symptomatic disease or the worsening of HIV-related symptoms is associated with depression and psychological distress; these were both cross-sectional and prospective studies involving gay men, men with haemophilia and heterosexual men and women (Catalán, Burgess and Klimes, 1995; McClure *et al.*, 1996; Lyketsos *et al.*, 1996a; Catalán *et al.*, 1996; Siegel, Karus and Raveis, 1997; Griffin *et al.*, 1998). Other findings are rare exceptions (Rabkin *et al.*, 1997). It is easy to understand that for many individuals who had succeeded in their efforts to adjust to being HIV positive and had developed ways of coping with their asymptomatic status, the onset of the first episode of illness or the presence of troublesome symptoms indicating disease progression would act as a precipitant of severe psychological morbidity. Disfiguring conditions, such as facial Kaposi's sarcoma, or conditions causing severe functional limitation, such as CMV (cytomegalovirus) retinitis, are particularly likely to cause difficulties.

Personality Factors

In general, individuals with personality difficulties or personality disorders are less likely to cope well with adversity, and as a result are at greater risk of developing mood disorders and other mental problems, and this is also true in the case of HIV infection, where studies have described this association both in cross-sectional and longitudinal designs. There is also some evidence to suggest that people with personality disorders, in particular those with borderline or antisocial personality disorders are at greater risk of acquiring HIV infection (Johnson *et al.*, 1995; Golding and Perkins, 1996; Johnson *et al.*, 1996). Ways of coping with difficulties tend to be a reflection of personality traits, and cross-sectional studies have shown how the use of avoidance, mental and behavioural disengagement, helplessness, denial and decreased use of fighting spirit are associated with greater psychological morbidity (Kurdek and Siesky, 1990; Leserman, Perkins and Evans, 1992; Catalán, Burgess and Klimes, 1995).

Past Psychiatric History

Individuals who prior to acquiring HIV infection have received in- or outpatient psychiatric care are at greater risk of developing mental health problems following infection (Dew, Ragni and Nimorwicz, 1990; Catalán *et al.*, 1992a,b), suggesting the presence of a personal vulnerability to adversity. In some instances, personality difficulties or personality disorder will have been implicated in the psychiatric contact. Substance misuse may also be relevant (see below), as may be social and relationship factors.

Social Support and Other Factors

In general, good social supports and the presence of confiding relationships have been shown to be associated with a lower prevalence of psychological morbidity, and this finding applies to people with HIV infection as well, so that HIV individuals lacking in adequate social supports usually report greater levels of psychological distress (Nott, Vedhara and Power, 1995; Catalán, Burgess and Klimes, 1995; Catalán *et al.*, 1996; Katz *et al.*, 1996; McClure *et al.*, 1996; Siegel, Karus and Raveis, 1997).

Adverse Life Events

Events with a negative impact appear to be associated with the development of psychological morbidity in people with HIV infection, and it has been argued that severe life stress might have a possible adverse role in HIV disease progression (Evans *et al.*, 1997) (see Chapter 11 for a discussion of psychoimmunology and HIV infection research). A particular adverse life event faced by many people with HIV infection is the experience of deaths due to AIDS among partners and friends (Viney *et al.*, 1992; Catalán, Burgess and Klimes, 1995). Multiple bereavements, loss of social supports, survivor's guilt, and concerns about one's own health can conspire to make what is already a difficult situation, extremely hard to cope with, leading to unresolved and complex grief reactions (Sherr *et al.*, 1992; Wright and Coyle, 1996; Gluhoski, Fishman and Perry, 1997).

Personal and Demographic Characteristics

While there is no compelling evidence that age is a predictive factor for emotional distress in people with HIV, it has been suggested that older individuals are at greater risk for psychiatric disorders, in particular those related to cognitive impairment and dementia (Catalán, Burgess and Klimes, 1995; Meadows, Le Marechal and Catalán, 1998). 'Brain reserve', a concept that refers to IQ and educational attainments, has been connected with the risk of developing HIV-related cognitive impairment (Stern *et al.*, 1996). Injecting drug users, as opposed to other HIV transmission categories, have the poorest psychological status, often having experienced social and psychological difficulties prior to acquiring the infection (Gala *et al.*, 1993), and with persistent drug use contributing to the problems in view of its inadequacy as a coping mechanism. Gender and ethnicity may also play a part.

A number of studies have suggested that women suffer more HIV-related emotional distress, and that women in developed countries seem to have worse access to medical services than men, which may have adverse effects also on their general physical health (Catalán, Burgess and Klimes, 1995;

Kennedy *et al.*, 1995). In developed countries, ethnicity appears to be a predictor of psychological disturbance in HIV, US Hispanic gay men and Black Americans showing greater emotional distress and lesser social supports than White men (Mays and Cochran, 1987; Ceballos-Capitaine *et al.*, 1990; Ostrow *et al.*, 1991; Spalding, 1995).

Mental Health Problems at the Time of HIV Testing

Psychological Status of People Seeking HIV Testing

Routine laboratory testing for HIV antibodies has been available to clinicians since 1985, while viral load tests entered clinical practice in 1996. Prior to 1985 it was possible to be concerned about being infected even in the absence of HIV-related symptoms, but there was no definite proof of infection until specific illnesses developed. Thus people who in those days regarded themselves as being at risk of AIDS, sometimes with very good reasons for their fear, were called 'worried well' (Forstein, 1984; Morin, Charles and Malyon, 1984), a term subsequently used in a different and somewhat inaccurate way to describe people who remain fearful of having HIV infection in spite of one or more HIV negative test results.

Concerns about HIV infection in spite of negative test results and adequate counselling should be regarded as a *symptom*, rather than a diagnosis, as such health worries can be part of a wide range of psychiatric disorders, including adjustment, obsessional and somatization disorders, hypochondriasis, and delusional disorders such as schizophrenia or severe affective illness. Careful assessment is therefore essential before applying the label 'worried well' to people with persistent worries involving HIV infection (Catalán, Burgess and Klimes, 1995).

Official guidelines endorsed by the World Health Organization (WHO) and other statutory and voluntary organizations stress that HIV testing should only be carried out with the individual's informed consent, except in exceptional circumstances. Pre-test counselling or discussion should involve the provision of information about HIV transmission, the significance of a positive and negative result, and discussion of the person's concerns. This task requires knowledge and skills of the kind that all health care workers should possess, and there has been in recent years a move away from regarding pre-test counselling as something that only specialists should undertake (Miller and Lipman, 1996).

Similarly, as the development of new treatments against HIV has gathered pace and the advantages of early HIV diagnosis and treatment become more apparent, HIV testing has begun to be perceived in a different light, less as the start of a death sentence, and more as the opportunity for access to effective treatment. Note that much of the research on the psychological consequences of HIV testing was carried out before the new anti-HIV treatments were introduced, at a time when there were far fewer therapeutic options available; it is likely that people seeking voluntary testing today differ from earlier individuals both in terms of their personal characteristics and their expectations. Uptake of HIV in clinical settings shows a wide range of rates of acceptance (Irwin, Valdiserri and Homberg, 1996) as does the positivity rate (Birthisle *et al.*, 1996).

Clinical experience suggests that people seeking HIV testing present with mild to moderate levels of distress. Following pre-test counselling some will decide against testing, presumably reassured about their low risk of infection. Among those who undergo testing, the results will predictably influence their subsequent emotional status. In a New York study of people seeking testing for HIV, Perry *et al.* (1990) reported on the psychiatric status of 200 individuals, including gay and bisexual men, injecting drug users, and non-drug-using heterosexual men and women. At the time of testing, subjects were no more psychologically disturbed than would have been expected in a comparable community sample, but they had much higher rates of past psychopathology than expected: a history of mood disorders, in particular depression, was present in 40 per cent, while 30 per cent had a history of substance misuse. Interestingly, those who were subsequently found to be HIV positive did not differ from negatives in their mental health at the time of testing or in the past. One important implication of these results, which have been replicated elsewhere, is the possible effect of a past history of mental health problems on the risk of developing further psychological difficulties in those found to be HIV positive.

In a separate report, Perry, Jacobsberg and Fishman (1990) found that 30 per cent of those seeking testing disclosed suicidal ideas during pre-test counselling. A week after notification of the results, there was no change for HIV positives, while in negatives the proportion with persistent suicidal ideas had been reduced almost by one-half. Two months later and after post-test counselling, about 15 per cent had suicidal ideas regardless of their serostatus (see Chapter 6 for a review of suicidal behaviour in HIV).

Psychological Status after HIV Testing

Notification of a positive test result is usually associated with severe, if transient, distress. Occasionally the reaction may be extreme, the person requiring intense support. Early research in the United States showed that people who chose to be given the result of a positive test reported declining psychological health during follow-up, while those who did not know their positivity showed improvement over the same period. Seronegatives, regardless of whether they knew their results, improved over time (Ostrow *et al.*, 1989).

Later studies give a somewhat different picture. London researchers studied newly diagnosed individuals, and found no differences in levels of psychological distress between HIV positives and negatives when they presented for testing (and did not know their serostatus) and at 6 and 12 months after being told the results (Riccio *et al.*, 1993; Pugh *et al.*, 1994). Similar findings were reported by Perry *et al.* (1993) in New York, who at 12 months after notification of the result found no differences in psychological morbidity between positives and negatives. The finding that seropositive individuals in the more recent studies had no worse psychological status than negatives at follow-up appears at first contrary to expectation. However, note that in both studies patients had received pre- and post-test counselling, and by then both London and New York had well-developed peer group support networks, which arguably could have contributed to the favourable outcome. It is also quite possible that seropositive individuals experienced more psychological distress immediately following notification, distress which abated by the time the 6 and 12 month follow-up assessments took place.

In summary, systematic research does confirm that for the majority of individuals the psychological distress associated with notification of a positive test result is of mild to moderate severity and of limited duration. This is not to say that no individual suffers major psychological distress, but rather that such cases are relatively rare. A group of individuals at risk of psychological problems following testing includes those who discover their serostatus when they develop symptomatic disease, in particular if the person had suspected the possibility of infection but used avoidance as a coping strategy (Katz, 1992). HIV testing at the time of symptomatic disease is relatively common, particularly when the infection has been acquired through heterosexual contact (Beevor and Catalán, 1993; Wortley *et al.*, 1995).

Mental Health Problems in Asymptomatic People with HIV

Following infection there is usually a fairly long period of asymptomatic HIV infection, lasting 10 years or more. However, this asymptomatic stage does show considerable variability in its length, and it is not always easy to predict the likelihood of progression, although there have been recent advances in this respect, based on the measurement of viral load and CD4 count (CD4 cells are a type of lymphocyte; they are also called helper T cells). Furthermore, the seroconversion date is seldom known with accuracy, and in a substantial proportion of individuals the diagnosis of HIV infection is made shortly before or at the time when symptoms develop, giving little time to adjust to the new situation without suffering other health problems. For many people living with HIV, this period of respite and good health is a very important one, allowing the person to attempt to come to terms with the diagnosis, reassess his or her life, clarify priorities and make decisions. Anticipated losses, such as those affecting health and physical independence, employment, self-esteem, support of family and friends, and future, among many others will need attention (Kalichman, 1995). While many people living with HIV will negotiate these difficulties successfully, not everyone will be able to cope effectively;

unresolved issues may become prominent again, or current stressors may add to the burden, as discussed in the earlier section on HIV and development of mental health disorders.

Research Evidence

Much empirical research has been carried out on the psychological status and problems of people with HIV infection, including those at different stages of infection, and reviews of this extensive literature are available (Kalichman and Sikkema, 1994; Catalán, Burgess and Klimes, 1995; Kalichman, 1995; Lyketsos and Federman, 1995; Rabkin, 1996; Fishman, Lyketsos and Treisman, 1996). Here is a summary of the key findings; the full coverage can be found in the review material quoted above.

There are complex methodological problems involved when attempting to answer what may seem a simple question, including well-known obstacles such as representativeness of the samples, nature of comparison groups, instruments used, subjects' HIV stage, design of the study, and the sample size. These difficulties go some way towards explaining some of the contradictory findings reported. Earlier studies tended to include gay and bisexual men only, but over the years there has been a gradual broadening of the range of subjects, and there are now reports that include men with haemophilia, injecting drug users and non-drug-using heterosexual men and women. Most reports, however, are from developed countries, and much remains to be learnt about the psychological impact of HIV in people from developing countries.

The large majority of studies of HIV asymptomatics with an appropriate seronegative comparison group find very few differences in distress and psychological status between the two groups. A few studies do report somewhat worse symptoms in positives, but the opposite is also true in a small number of studies. While this conclusion may seem surprising at first, it is relevant to remember that the impact of notification of seropositivity tends to be time-limited, helped by the absence of physical symptoms. Another factor may be the nature of the seronegative controls: in spite of their HIV status, they tend to have the same prevalence of past psychopathology as the positives, and so carry a comparable risk of further mental health problems.

Levels of psychological distress in individuals who regard themselves at risk of infection and who seek testing, regardless of their HIV status, are generally low, although possibly a little higher than would be expected in demographically comparable community samples. HIV asymptomatic seropositives represent a minority (between 12 and 30 per cent) of all HIV patients referred to general hospital-based mental health services, the majority being symptomatics (Sno, Storosum and Swinkels, 1989; Ayuso Mateos *et al.*, 1989; Seth *et al.*, 1991). Common diagnoses given to asymptomatic individuals referred to mental health services are adjustment disorder, major depression and other forms of depression, substance misuse, panic disorder, personality problems and sexual dysfunction. Organic brain syndromes (acute and chronic) and new onset psychotic illnesses are very rare in this group of patients.

Mental Health Problems in Symptomatic People with HIV

The terminology used to describe HIV symptomatic disease has changed over the years, and while some labels have become obsolete, such as ARC or PGL, others have proved more resilient, in particular the term AIDS. In so far as AIDS is an operationally defined concept, arrived at by the development of a so-called AIDS-defining illness, and therefore with a clear boundary to separate it from non-AIDS, it is easy to see its appeal, particularly for those who have not yet reached the dreaded stage, and could thus see themselves as being 'only HIV'. Conversely, an AIDS diagnosis could bring with it more than just a label or a collection of unpleasant symptoms: a new identity would be part of the package, including feelings of gloom about the future, fears of social rejection and awareness of approaching death.

It is well known that medical terms have a social and psychological meaning of their own, beyond their strictly descriptive sense, and this is especially true when dealing with diseases which carry strong stigma, such as tuberculosis (TB), sexually transmitted diseases or cancer (Sontag, 1991). It is difficult to imagine the disappearence of the term AIDS, but there is no doubt that since 1996 its significance has changed; people with HIV and their doctors are giving more attention to better indicators of prognosis, such as viral load levels and CD4 count. Whether or not someone has an AIDS diagnosis may turn out to be less important than the amount of HIV detectable in serum and the degree of immunosuppression. This section summarizes the mental health problems of people with what used to be known as ARC (AIDS-related complex) and is now called symptomatic or advanced HIV infection and AIDS. Review papers and resource books should be consulted for more detail.

Research Evidence

There are fewer systematic studies involving symptomatic individuals, but research findings are in general more consistent when dealing with this group. The majority of surveys have found higher levels of anxiety, depression and other psychological symptoms in symptomatic individuals compared with negative controls, or with asymptomatics. Interestingly, non-AIDS symptomatic disease or ARC is reported in some cases to be associated with worse psychological status than AIDS (Perry and Markowitz, 1986; Tross *et al.*, 1987). In general, surveys of gay and bisexual men and surveys of men with haemophilia have tended to find worse psychological status in symptomatics, whereas studies of injecting drug users or mixed populations are less likely to find differences (Lyketsos *et al.*, 1996b). There is litle research on non-drug-using heterosexual men and women, and results are mixed.

Among HIV patients referred to the mental health services, symptomatics represent the majority of referrals (Bialer *et al.*, 1996). Early surveys suggested that between 20 and 30 per cent of medical inpatients with AIDS were referred for psychiatric assessment, most suffering from depression (Perry and Tross, 1984; Dilley *et al.*, 1985). Later studies have tended to report rates of referral among symptomatics of around 15 per cent (Buhrich and Cooper, 1987). While reported rates give some idea of the degree of need, it is not possible to generalize from these figures, as referral to psychiatric services is influenced by many factors, including not just the degree of psychological distress experienced by patients, but also the threshold for recognition of such disturbance by doctors and others, and availability of services to which to refer patients.

Common diagnoses in symptomatics will include organic brain syndromes, both dementia and delirium, major depression, problems related to substance misuse, problems adjusting to declining health, and problems with relatives and partners. Bialer *et al.* (1996) compared people with AIDS referred to a general hospital psychiatric service with non-HIV patients referred to the same service, and they found a significant excess of dementia in the AIDS group, but lower rates of substance misuse, major depression and personality disorder.

Palliative Care

In the final stages of HIV infection there is often an increase in neuropsychiatric and other mental health problems, partly as a result of brain impairment, but also due to the general loss of independence and autonomy that declining health usually brings. The difference between understandable, normal sadness or fear of the future, and pathological syndromes or symptoms can be difficult to make, although in practice palliation of distress and discomfort will be the principal aim, regardless of their causes. Much of what has been published in relation to palliative care is based on the experiences of people with cancer (Kubler-Ross, 1970; Parkes, 1986; Vachon, 1993), but there is now a growing literature concerning people with HIV (Sims and Moss, 1991; Catania *et al.*, 1992; Passik *et al.*, 1995; Kaldjian, Jekel and Friedland, 1998).

In a London survey of the place of death for people with AIDS (Guthrie, Nelson and Gazzard, 1996), the authors reported a change from the early days of the epidemic when most died in hospital, to the 1990s when less than half did so, 30 per cent dying at home and 20 per cent in hospices. Interestingly, almost two-thirds of deaths occurred in the place where the person had intended to die, unplanned deaths being usually the result of sudden and unexpected deterioration leading to hospitalization. While care in hospice is likely to be better tailored to the needs of terminally ill people, in practice only a minority of people with AIDS die in them, so it is important to ensure the emotional and practical needs of terminally ill people with AIDS are met whether they are in hospital or at home, possibly using imaginative primary care based appoaches (Butters and Higginson, 1995; Koffman, Higginson and Naysmith, 1996).

It has been shown that terminally ill people with AIDS feel less hopeful than similarly ill patients with cancer (Herth, 1990), possibly because of fears of rejection and isolation. Baker and Seager (1991) compared the needs of hospice residents with and without AIDS, and found AIDS patients to have fewer community supports and require more hospice staff involvement than other patients. In contrast, Catania *et al.* (1992) found that disease progression was associated with increased involvement with the individual's biological family and with a reduction in death-related anxiety, leading to better communication and support from parents and other relatives.

There are few systematic studies of the mental health problems that arise in the final stages of AIDS, but there are valuable descriptions of the emotional, social, spiritual and physical needs that can occur (Sims and Moss, 1991). Organic brain syndromes are very common, particularly delirium, but also depressive syndromes, behavioural problems and psychotic episodes (Catalán, Burgess and Klimes, 1995).

Impact of Long-Term Survival

Even before the introduction of new treatments, it was known that a proportion of people with HIV infection had good prognosis, showing extended survival and minimal change in immune function and health over a long period of time (Buchbinder *et al.*, 1994). The reasons were unclear for the good outcome of non-progressors (generally asymptomatic) or long-term survivors (after symptomatic disease), but they were thought to include biological factors, such as HIV strain and load, genetic factors in the infected individual, treatment, and lifestyle and psychological factors (Easterbrook, 1994).

The possible contribution to survival of psychological factors, including personality, life events, ways of coping and social supports, was the subject of much interest, and there was evidence that non-progressors regard mental attitude as the most important factor in their good health (Troop *et al.*, 1997). In a study of long-term survivors, including 53 gay men who had AIDS for more than three years, Remien, Rabkin and Williams (1992) reported the use of a wide range of coping strategies, such as active coping, taking control of their health, the pursuit of pleasurable activities, and making good use of social supports. Low levels of psychological morbidity and no suicide attempts following HIV diagnosis were reported by Rabkin *et al.* (1993) in a study of 60 gay men with a diagnosis of AIDS for at least three years, although as many as one-third had wanted to die at some stage after their diagnosis, and one-quarter considered suicide as a future option.

There are complex methodological problems involved in research that attempts to demonstrate a relationship between psychological variables and survival, and positive evidence is poor or absent (Keet *et al.*, 1994; Veugelers *et al.*, 1994; Munoz *et al.*, 1995); see Chapter 11 for a discussion of the broader issue of psychoimmunological factors in HIV). It is true that many long-term survivors coped reasonably well, maintaining a sense of mastery and low levels of stress. But others found that the years took their toll, years of awareness about their status, uncertainty over the future, changes in employment and career, exposure to multiple deaths and loss of significant others, and concerns about treatment decisions; and they experienced the range of psychological problems described for the HIV symptomatic individuals.

In recent years, however, the situation has changed dramatically. The introduction of protease inhibitors in combination with other antiretrovirals early in 1996, known as highly active antiretroviral therapy (HAART), has had a striking effect on HIV-related morbidity and mortality (Sepkowitz, 1998). In parallel with improvements in health and increased survival, the new treatment regimes have shown substantial reductions in plasma viral load below detectable levels accompanied by increases in CD4 count, leading to the expectation that the virus could be totally eradicated, in spite of calls for caution (Grant and Abrams, 1998). People with advanced HIV infection and troublesome symptoms treated with the new regimes have shown substantial improvement in their quality of life and ability to function, and often in their mental attitude and levels of stress. For some, however, unexpected improvements in health and the prospect of longer survival have not been free from difficulties. While little systematic empirical research is available, preliminary reports (Anderson and Weatherburn, 1998) and clinical experience have highlighted some common areas of difficulty.

Readjusting to Extended Life Expectancy

The majority of people who have known about their HIV infection for some years have developed a way of dealing with a reduced expectation of survival and with the limitations their health has placed on their lives. Symptomatic individuals in particular will have reconsidered their career, relationships and long-term plans, and a proportion will need to depend on state benefits, their families and friends. The result of new treatments will usually lead to a re-examination of existential and practical issues that had been dealt with before, but now from a new perspective. Some will find this process painless and straightforward; others will find that coming to terms with the real possibility of having a long-term future leads to difficult decisions about relationships, work, financial matters, etc. (Hirschel and Francioli, 1998). The development of what has been termed a 'second life' agenda (Rabkin and Ferrando, 1997) will not be a painless process for many individuals.

Uncertainty about the Long-Term Benefits of Treatment

The term 'Lazarus effect' has been used to describe the recent phenomenon of people with AIDS rising from their deathbeds, if not their tombs, thanks to the new combination therapies. Perhaps a more appropriate story is the Ancient Greek myth of Orpheus and his wife Eurydike. Eurydike was sent to Hades, and Orpheus was only permitted to bring her back from the Underworld by charming the gods with his singing. But on the journey he broke his promise not to look round to see Eurydike following, and so on the way back to life, Orpheus lost her forever. To engineer a happy ending, operatic versions include a further rescue by the gods.

Many people with HIV have been through false dawns before, have learnt of the development of drug resistance, and have known people who have not responded to the new treatments (Fatkenheuer *et al.*, 1997). Against this knowledge, not everyone will find it easy to give themselves permision to think and plan in the long-term, to consider giving up state benefits, start a new career or commit themselves to a relationship. For some, improvement in health may be seen as a brief respite, a last chance to lead a normal life before the inevitable decline, resulting in a desperate effort to cram activities, achievement and pleasure into what is feared to be a brief period of time. Others may become intensely proccupied with minute variations in their viral load or obsessed with reaching undetectable levels (Hirschel and Francioni, 1998).

Treatment Adherence

It is not easy to take medication regularly and for long periods of time, especially if the regime is complicated, the tablets are many, side effects occur, and the process reminds the person of their illness. Not everyone is able to adhere to the treatment regime perfectly, and a number of factors have been identified, such as demographic, psychosocial, medication-related and health care delivery variables (Mehta, Moore and Graham, 1997). Unfortunately, in the case of highly active antiretroviral therapy (HAART), less than perfect adherence to treatment can result in the development of drug-resistant strains of the virus and lead to viral breakthrough (Carpenter *et al.*, 1997), sometimes even after a week of missed medication or 80 per cent adherence (Roberts, 1995; Condra *et al.*, 1995; Jacobsen *et al.*, 1996).

Recent surveys in the United States using self-report questionnaires, which may give a somewhat rosier picture of what is actually happening, have suggested that as many as 30 per cent had missed at least one dose in the previous three days (Hecht *et al.*, 1998) and 36 per cent in the last two weeks (Chesney and Ickovics, 1997). Others have found even more worrying levels of adherence (Weiss, 1998). Reasons given for missing doses include forgetting to take the tablets, being away from home or busy with other activities, medication side effects, and depressed mood (Chesney and Ickovics, 1997; Hecht *et al.*, 1998). Missing doses was also associated with a higher regular intake of alcohol (Chesney and Ickovics, 1997). Adverse side effects of medication, in particular those with cosmetic consequences, may affect compliance (Lipsky, 1998). Efforts are being made to develop effective ways of increasing treatment adherence to the new combination therapies (Chesney and Hecht, 1998).

Normalization of Emotional and Sexual Relationships

Acknowledging the possibility of having a long-term future will also open up options regarding relationships. Some will give further consideration to the chances of having children and the risks of the baby being born with HIV infection, and this process may involve agonizing decisions. Those who are not in a relationship may seek to become involved again, and issues concerned with how much and when to self-disclose will need to be examined. People with HIV who have lost a partner to AIDS sometimes find it particularly difficult to think seriously about further relationships, among other reasons, for fear of putting the new partner through the experience of having to take care of someone dying of AIDS, and such fears are not easily dispelled by improvement in health.

Sexual dysfunction problems can become a source of concern when someone who has lost interest in sex when very unwell, now begins to attempt to re-establish sexual relations but experiences problems of arousal or orgasm. Sexual dysfunctions are common in people with HIV infection, particularly in symptomatic disease, and their causes are complex, but there are ways of helping individuals and couples with such problems (Catalán, Burgess and Klimes, 1995; Sellmeyer and Grunfeld, 1996). Restoration of sexual function can raise concerns about the risk of sexual transmission of HIV to others.

Changing Social and Personal Significance of HIV Infection

The way HIV infection is socially perceived is begining to change from a stigmatizing 'plague' or 'death sentence' to a chronic treatable condition, like many other medical disorders. While these shifts in perception are in many ways positive, they can also bring about subtle changes in the way people with HIV see themselves and are viewed by others. Normalization of HIV may mean that some people with the infection who have developed a sense of identity through membership of the HIV community, begin now to feel disenfranchised and isolated, losing contact with support groups and organizations which are themselves trying to survive in a climate where they are not thought to be needed any more.

A 'sympathy fatigue' may start to emerge, so that those who felt they belonged to a charmed group are now expected to deal with problems and difficulties just like everyone else. The perception of HIV as a treatable condition may also bring about a weakening of the resolve to prevent the spread of infection: if HIV is not a death sentence, if it is like any other STD, why should we be so concerned about what is a relatively uncommon condition? Finally, a new version of survivor's guilt can arise in the wake of the new combination therapies: if only all those who have perished had had access to these new treatments! In the United States, Kobayashi (1997) has described perceptively the stages of adaptation to HIV and social responses from 1981 until the introduction of new combination treatments in 1997, highlighting the changes in the psychological responses to the epidemic.

References

ANDERSON, W. and WEATHERBURN, P. (1998) *The impact of combination therapy on the lives of people with HIV*, London: Sigma Research.

AYUSO MATEOS, J.L., BAYON PEREZ, C., STO DOMINGO CARRASCO, J. *et al.* (1989) 'Psychiatric aspects of patients with HIV infection in the general hospital', *Psychotherapy and psychosomatics*, **52**, pp. 110–13.

BAKER, N. and SEAGER, R. (1991) 'A comparison of the psychosocial needs of patients with AIDS and those with other diseases', *Hospice Journal*, **7**, pp. 61–69.

BEEVOR, A. and CATALÁN, J. (1993) 'Women's experience of HIV testing', *AIDS Care*, **5**, pp. 177–86.

BIALER, P.A., WALLACK, J.J., PRENZLAUER, S.L. *et al.* (1996) 'Psychiatric comorbidity among hospitalized AIDS patients vs. non-AIDS patients referred for psychiatric consultation', *Psychosomatics*, **37**, pp. 469–75.

BIRTHISLE, K., MAGUIRE, H., ATKINSON, P. *et al.* (1996) 'Who's having HIV tests? An audit of HIV test requests in a large London teaching hospital', *Health Trends*, **28**, pp. 60–63.

BUCHBINDER, S.P., KATZ, M.H., HESSOL, N.A. *et al.* (1994) 'Long-term HIV-1 infection without immunological progression', *AIDS*, **8**, pp. 1123–28.

BUHRICH, N. and COOPER, D. (1987) 'Requests for psychiatric consultation concerning 22 patients with AIDS and ARC', *Australia and New Zealand Journal of Psychiatry*, **21**, pp. 346–53.

BUTTERS, E. and HIGGINSON, I. (1995) 'Two HIV/AIDS community support teams: patient characteristics, problems at referral and during the last 6 weeks of life', *AIDS Care*, **7**, pp. 593–603.

CARPENTER, C.C.J., FISCHEL, M.A., HAMMER, S.M. *et al.* (1997) 'Antiretroviral therapy for HIV infection in 1997: Updated recommendations of the International AIDS Society–USA Panel', *Journal of the American Medical Association*, **277**, pp. 1962–69.

CATALÁN, J., BURGESS, A. and KLIMES, I. (1995) *Psychological medicine of HIV infection*, Oxford: Oxford University Press.

CATALÁN, J., KLIMES, I., DAY, A. *et al.* (1992a) 'The psychosocial impact of HIV infection in gay men: a controlled investigation and factors associated with psychiatric morbidity', *British Journal of Psychiatry*, **161**, pp. 774–78.

CATALÁN, J., KLIMES, I., BOND, A. *et al.* (1992b) 'The psychosocial impact of HIV infection in men with haemophilia: controlled investigation and factors associated with psychiatric morbidity', *Journal of Psychosomatic Research*, **36**, pp. 409–16.

CATALÁN, J., BEEVOR, A., CASSIDY, L. *et al.* (1996) 'Women and HIV infection: investigation of its psychological consequences', *Journal of Psychosomatic Research*, **41**, pp. 39–47.

CATANIA, J., TURNER, H., CHOI, K.H. *et al.* (1992) 'Coping with death anxiety: help-seeking and social support among gay men with various HIV diagnosis', *AIDS*, **6**, pp. 999–1005.

CEBALLOS-CAPITAINE, A., SZAPOCZNIC, J., BLANEY, N. *et al.* (1990) 'Ethnicity, emotional distress, stress-related disruption and coping among HIV positive gay males', *Hispanic Journal of Behavioral Sciences*, **12**, pp. 135–52.

CHESNEY, M.A. and HECHT, F.M. (1998) 'Adherence to HIV antiretroviral therapy: an essential element to understanding treatment effect', paper presented at the Second European Conference on the Methods and Results of Social and Behavioural Research on AIDS, Paris, 12–15, January.

CHESNEY, M. and ICKOVICS, J. for the Recruitment, Adherence and Retention Committe of the ACTG (1997) 'Adherence to combination therapy in AIDS clinical trials', paper presented at the Annual Meeting of the AIDS Clinical Trials Group, Washington DC, July.

CONDRA, J.H., SCHLEIF, W.A., BLAHY, O.M. *et al.* (1995) 'In vivo emergence of HIV-1 variants resistant to multiple protease inhibitors', *Nature*, **374**, pp. 569–71.

DAVIS, R.F., METZGER, D.S., MEYERS, K. *et al.* (1995) 'Long-term changes in psychological symptomatology associated with HIV serostatus among male injecting drug users', *AIDS*, **9**, pp. 73–79.

DEW, A., RAGNI, M. and NIMORWICZ, P. (1990) 'Infection, with HIV and vulnerability to psychiatric distress: a study of men with haemophilia', *Archives of General Psychiatry*, **47**, pp. 737–44.

DILLEY, J., OCHITILL, H., PERL, M. *et al.* (1985) 'Findings in psychiatric consultation with patients with AIDS', *American Journal of Psychiatry*, **142**, pp. 82–86.

EASTERBROOK, P. (1994) 'Non-progression in HIV infection', *AIDS*, **8**, pp. 1179–82.

EVANS, D.L., LESERMAN, J., PERKINS, D.O. *et al.* (1997) 'Severe life stress as a predictor of early disease progression in HIV infection', *American Journal of Psychiatry*, **154**, pp. 630–34.

FATKENHEUER, G., THEISEN, A., ROCKSTROH, J. *et al.* (1997) 'Virological treatment failure of protease inhibitor therapy in an unselected cohort of HIV-infected patients', *AIDS*, **11**, pp. F113–16.

FISHMAN, M., LYKETSOS, C.G. and TREISMAN, G. (1996) 'Mood disorders in HIV infection', *International Review of Psychiatry*, **8**, pp. 267–76.

FORSTEIN, M. (1984) 'AIDS anxiety in the worried well', in: Nichols, S. and Ostrow, D. (eds) *Psychiatric implications of AIDS*, Washington DC: American Psychiatric Press.

GALA, C., PERGAMI, A., CATALÁN, J. *et al.* (1993) 'The psychosocial impact of HIV infection in gay men, drug users and heterosexuals: a controlled investigation', *British Journal of Psychiatry*, **163**, pp. 651–59.

GLUHOSKI, V.L., FISHMAN, B. and PERRY, S.W. (1997) 'The impact of multiple bereavement in a gay male sample', *AIDS Education and Prevention*, **9**, 6, pp. 521–31.

GOLDING, M. and PERKINS, D.O. (1996) 'Personality disorder in HIV infection', *International Review of Psychiatry*, **8**, pp. 253–58.

GRANT, R.M. and ABRAMS, D.I. (1998) 'Not all is dead in HIV-1 graveyard', *Lancet*, **351**, pp. 308–9.

GRIFFIN, K.W., RABKIN, J., REMIEN, R. *et al.* (1998) 'Disease severity, physical limitations and depression in HIV infected men', *Journal of Psychosomatic Research*, **44**, pp. 219–27.

GUTHRIE, B., NELSON, M. and GAZZARD, B. (1996) 'Are people with HIV in London able to die where they plan?', *AIDS Care*, **8**, pp. 709–13.

HECHT, F.M., COLFAX, G., SWANSON, M. *et al.* (1998) 'Adherence and effectiveness of protease inhibitors in clinical practice', paper presented at the Fifth Conference on Retroviruses and Opportunistic Infections, Chicago IL, 2–6 February.

HERTH, K. (1990) 'Fostering hope in terminally ill people', *Journal of Advanced Nursing*, **15**, pp. 1250–59.

HIRSCHEL, B. and FRANCIONI, P. (1998) 'Progress and problems in the fight against AIDS', *New England Journal of Medicine*, **338**, pp. 906–8.

HOLT, R., COURT, P., VEDHARA, K. *et al.* (1998) 'The role of disclosure in coping with HIV infection', *AIDS Care*, **10**, pp. 49–60.

IRWIN, K.L., VALDISERRI, R.O. and HOLMBERG, S. (1996) 'The acceptability of voluntary HIV testing in the US: a decade of lessons learnt', *AIDS*, **10**, pp. 1707–17.

JACOBSEN, H., HANGGI, M., OTT, M. *et al.* (1996) 'In vivo resistance to an HIV-1 protease inhibitor: mutations, kinetics and frequencies', *Journal of Infectious Diseases*, **173**, pp. 1379–87.

JOHNSON, J.G., WILLIAMS, J., RABKIN, J. *et al.* (1995) 'Axis I psychiatric symptoms associated with HIV infection and personality disorder', *American Journal of Psychiatry*, **152**, pp. 551–54.

JOHNSON, J.G., WILLIAMS, J., GOETZ, R. *et al.* (1996) 'Personality disorders predict onset of axis I disorders and impaired functioning among homosexual men with and at risk of HIV infection', *Archives of General Psychiatry*, **53**, pp. 350–57.

KALDJIAN, L.C., JEKEL, J.F. and FRIEDLAND, G. (1998) 'End-of-life decisions in HIV-positive patients: the role of spiritual beliefs', *AIDS*, **12**, pp. 103–7.

KALICHMAN, S.C. (1995) *Understanding AIDS: a guide for mental health professionals*, Washington DC: American Psychological Association.

KALICHMAN, S.C. and SIKKEMA, K.J. (1994) 'Psychological sequelae of HIV infection and AIDS: review of empirical findings', *Clinical Psychology Review*, **14**, pp. 611–32.

KATZ, M. (1992) 'Coping with HIV: why people delay care', *Annals of Internal Medicine*, **117**, p. 797.

KATZ, M.H., DOUGLAS, J.M. JR, BOLAN, G.A. *et al.* (1996) 'Depression and use of mental health services among HIV-infected men', *AIDS Care*, **8**, pp. 433–42.

KEET, I.P., KROL, A., KLEIN, M.R. *et al.* (1994) 'Characteristics of long-term asymptomatic infection with HIV-1 in men with normal and low CD4 counts', *Journal of Infectious Diseases*, **169**, pp. 1236–43.

KENNEDY, C.A., SKURNICK, J.H., FOLEY, M. *et al.* (1995) 'Gender differences in HIV-related distress in heterosexual couples', *AIDS Care*, **7**, pp. s33–38.

KOBAYASHI, J.S. (1997) 'The evolution of adjustment issues in HIV/AIDS', *Bulletin of the Menninger Clinic*, **61**, pp. 146–88.

KOFFMAN, J., HIGGINSON, I. and NAYSMITH, A. (1996) 'Hospice at home – a new service for patients with advanced HIV/AIDS: a pilot evaluation of referrals and outcomes', *British Journal of General Practice*, **46**, pp. 539–40.

KUBLER-ROSS, E. (1970) *On Death and Dying*, London: Tavistock.

KURDEK, L. and SIESKY, G. (1990) 'The nature and correlates of psychological adjustment in gay men with AIDS-related conditions', *Journal of Applied Social Psychology*, **20**, pp. 846–60.

LESERMAN, J., PERKINS, D. and EVANS, D. (1992) 'Coping with the threat of AIDS', *American Journal of Psychiatry*, **149**, pp. 1514–20.

LIPSKY, J. (1998) 'Abnormal fat accumulation in patients with HIV-1 infection', *Lancet*, **351**, pp. 847–48.

LYKETSOS, C.G. and FEDERMAN, E.B. (1995) 'Psychiatric disorders and HIV infection: impact on one another', *Epidemiological Review*, **17**, pp. 152–64.

LYKETSOS, C.G., HOOVER, D.R., GUCCIONE, M. *et al.* (1996a) 'Changes in depressive symptoms as AIDS develops', *American Journal of Psychiatry*, **153**, pp. 1430–37.

LYKETSOS, C.G., HUTTON, H., FISHMAN, M. *et al.* (1996b) 'Psychiatric morbidity on entry to an HIV primary care clinic', *AIDS*, **10**, pp. 1033–39.

MCCLURE, J.B., CATZ, S., PREJEAN, J. *et al.* (1996) 'Factors associated with depression in a heterogeneous HIV-infected sample', *Journal of Psychosomatic Research*, **40**, pp. 407–15.

MAYS, V. and COCHRAN, S. (1987) 'AIDS and Black Americans: especial psychosocial issues', *Public Health Reports*, **102**, pp. 224–31.

MEADOWS, J., LE MARECHAL, K. and CATALÁN, J. (1998) 'Mental health problems in older adults with HIV referred to a psychological medicine unit', *AIDS Care*, **10**, pp. s105–12.

MEHTA, S., MOORE, R.D. and GRAHAM, N.M.H. (1997) 'Potential factors affecting adherence with HIV therapy', *AIDS*, **11**, pp. 1665–70.

MILLER, R. and LIPMAN, M. (1996) 'HIV pre-test discussion', *British Medical Journal*, **313**, p. 130.

MORIN, S., CHARLES, K. and MALYON, A. (1984) 'The psychological impact of AIDS on gay men', *American Psychologist*, **39**, pp. 1288–93.

MUNOZ, A., KIRBY, A.J., HE, Y.D. *et al.* (1995) 'Long-term survivors with HIV-1 infection: incubation period and longitudinal pattern of CD4 lymphocytes', *Journal of AIDS and Human Retrovirology*, **8**, pp. 495–505.

NOTT, K.H., VEDHARA, K. and POWER, M.J. (1995) 'The role of social support in HIV infection', *Psychological Medicine*, **25**, pp. 971–83.

OSTROW, D.G., JOSEPH, J., KESSLER, R. *et al.* (1989) 'Disclosure of HIV antibody status: behavioural and mental correlates', *AIDS Education and Prevention*, **1**, pp. 1–11.

OSTROW, D.G., WHITAKER, R., FRASIER, K. *et al.* (1991) 'Racial differences in social support and mental health in men with HIV infection: a pilot study', *AIDS Care*, **3**, pp. 55–62.

PARKES, C.M. (1986) 'Care of the dying: the role of the psychiatrist', *British Journal of Hospital Medicine*, **36**, pp. 250–55.

PASSIK, S.D., MCDONALD, M.V., ROSENFELD, B.D. *et al.* (1995) 'End of life issues in patients with AIDS: clinical and research considerations', *Journal of Pharmaceutical Care in Pain and Symptom Control*, **3**, pp. 91–111.

PERGAMI, A., CATALÁN, J., HULME, N. *et al.* (1994) 'How should a positive test be given? The patients view', *AIDS Care*, **6**, pp. 21–27.

PERRY, S. and MARKOWITZ, J. (1986) 'Psychiatric interventions for AIDS-spectrum disorders', *Hospital and Community Psychology*, **37**, pp. 1001–6.

PERRY, S. and TROSS, S. (1984) 'Psychiatric problems of AIDS in-patients at the New York hospital: preliminary report', *Public Health Reports*, **99**, pp. 201–5.

PERRY, S., JACOBSBERG, L. and FISHMAN, B. (1990) 'Suicidal ideation and HIV testing', *Journal of the American Medical Association*, **263**, pp. 679–82.

PERRY, S., JACOBSBERG, L., FISHMAN, B. *et al.* (1990) 'Psychiatric diagnosis before serological testing for HIV', *American Journal of Psychiatry*, **147**, pp. 89–93.

PERRY, S., JACOBSBERG, L., CARD, C. *et al.* (1993) 'Severity of psychiatric symptoms after HIV testing', *American Journal of Psychiatry*, **150**, pp. 775–79.

PUGH, K., RICCIO, M., JADRESIC, D. *et al.* (1994) 'A longitudinal study of the neuropsychiatric consequences of HIV-1 infection in gay men: psychosocial and health status at baseline and 12 month follow-up', *Psychological Medicine*, **24**, pp. 897–904.

RABKIN, J.G. (1996) 'Prevalence of psychiatric disorders in HIV illness', *International Review of Psychiatry*, **8**, pp. 157–66.

RABKIN, J.G. and FERRANDO, S. (1997) 'A "second life" agenda', *Archives of General Psychiatry*, **54**, pp. 1049–53.

RABKIN, J.G., REMIEN, R., KATOFF, L. *et al.* (1993) 'Suicidality in AIDS long-term survivors: what is the evidence?', *AIDS Care*, **5**, pp. 401–11.

RABKIN, J.G., GOETZ, R.R., REMIEN, R.H. *et al.* (1997) 'Stability of mood despite HIV illness progression in a group of homosexual men', *American Journal of Psychiatry*, **154**, pp. 231–38.

REMIEN, R.H., RABKIN, J. and WILLIAMS, J. (1992) 'Coping strategies and health beliefs of AIDS long-term survivors', *Psychology and Health*, **6**, pp. 335–45.

RICCIO, M., PUGH, K., JADRESIC, D. *et al.* (1993) 'Neuropsychiatric aspects of HIV-1 infection in gay men: controlled investigation of psychiatric, neuropsychiatric and neurological status', *Journal of Psychosomatic Research*, **37**, pp. 819–30.

ROBERTS, N.A. (1995) 'Drug resistance patterns of sequinavir and other protease inhibitors', *AIDS*, **9**, pp. s27–32.

SELLMEYER, D.E. and GRUNFELD, C. (1996) 'Endocrine and metabolic disturbances in HIV and AIDS', *Endocrine Reviews*, **17**, pp. 518–32.

SEPKOWITZ, K.A. (1998) 'Effect of HAART on natural history of AIDS-related opportunistic disorder', *Lancet*, **351**, pp. 228–30.

SETH, R., GRANVILLE-GROSSMAN, K., GOLDMEIER, D. *et al.* (1991) 'Psychiatric illness in patients with HIV infection and AIDS referred to the liaison psychiatrist', *British Journal of Psychiatry*, **159**, pp. 347–50.

SHERR, L., HEDGE, B., STEINHART, K. *et al.* (1992) 'Unique patterns of bereavement in HIV: implications for counselling', *Genitourinary Medicine*, **68**, pp. 378–81.

SIEGEL, K., KARUS, D. and RAVEIS, V, (1997) 'Correlates of change in depressive symptomatology among gay men with AIDS', *Health Psychology*, **16**, pp. 230–38.

SIMS, R. and MOSS, V. (1991) *Terminal Care for People with AIDS*, London: Edward Arnold.

SNO, H., STOROSUM, J. and SWINKELS, J. (1989) 'HIV infection: psychiatric findings in the Netherlands', *British Journal of Psychiatry*, **155**, pp. 814–17.

SONTAG, S. (1988) *AIDS and its Metaphors*, London: Penguin.

SPALDING, A.D. (1995) 'Racial minorities and other high-risk groups with HIV and AIDS at increased risk for psychological adjustment problems in association with health locus of control orientation', *Social Work in Health Care*, **21**, pp. 81–114.

STERN, R., SILVA, S., CHAISSON, N. *et al.* (1996) 'Influence of cognitive reserve on neuropsychological functioning in asymptomatic HIV-1 infection', *Archives of Neurology*, **53**, pp. 148–53.

TROOP, M., EASTERBROOK, P., THORNTON, S. *et al.* (1997) 'Reasons given by patients for non-progression in HIV infection', *AIDS Care*, **9**, pp. 133–42.

TROSS, S., HIRSCH, D., RABKIN, B. *et al.* (1987) 'Determinants of current psychiatric disorder in AIDS-spectrum patients', paper presented at the Third International Conference on AIDS, Washington DC.

VACHON, M. (1993) 'Emotional problems in palliative medicine', in: Doyle, D.,

Hanks, G. and MacDonald, N. (eds) *Oxford Textbook of Palliative Medicine*, Oxford: Oxford University Press.

VEUGELERS, P., PAGE, K., TINDALL, B. *et al.* (1994) 'Determinants of disease progression among homosexual men registered in the Tricontinental Seroconverter Study', *American Journal of Epidemiology*, **140**, pp. 747–58.

VINEY, L., HENRY, R., WALKER, B. *et al.* (1992) 'The psychosocial impact of multiple deaths from AIDS', *Omega*, **24**, pp. 151–63.

WEISS, J.J. (1998) 'Attitudinal factors relating to protease inhibitor therapy', paper presented at the Second European Conference on the Methods and Results of Social and Behavioural Research on AIDS, Paris, 12–15 January.

WORTLEY, P.M., CHU, S.Y., DIAZ, T. *et al.* (1995) 'HIV testing patterns: where, why, and when were persons with AIDS tested for HIV?', *AIDS*, **9**, pp. 487–92.

WRIGHT, C. and COYLE, A. (1996) 'Experiences of AIDS-related bereavement among gay men: implications for care', *Mortality*, **1**, pp. 267–82.

Chapter 3

HIV Disease and Its Impact on the Mental Health of Children

Lorraine Sherr

The mental health effects of HIV in children are profound. They raise a complex web of issues about emotional and physical well-being, often with no precedent in the literature for guidance or theory. This chapter introduces the issue of children and HIV, it briefly discusses the important role of vertical transmission, and it examines the factors of diagnosis, treatment, illness progression and survival. This serves as a background to the detailed exploration of the neurological and cognitive implications in developing children. There are systematic methodological problems in considering these issues, and they are explored in relation to investigations, studies and findings. Towards the end of the chapter, there is a detailed discussion on mother and family effects, behavioural problems in the presence of HIV and AIDS, and emotional and psychological consequences. By focusing on parents, siblings, grandparents and wider family members, the final section aims to provide some insight into mental health considerations for infected and uninfected children in families where HIV is present.

Background

There is a growing understanding of HIV infection in children. Much of this information is gathered in pursuance of a greater understanding of vertical transmission of HIV. Relatively less is known on the impact of HIV in adolescents, even though the majority of people who have AIDS in their twenties were probably infected as teenagers. Mental health is a broad concept and is often used to incorporate cognitive problems, emotional parameters and daily functioning. All these are important aspects for understanding HIV in children. Surprisingly they are often overlooked, with many workers focusing simply on the end of life, grief and death as the only mental health challenge for young children (Mok and Newell, 1995). Although end-of-life aspects are important, and are briefly discussed, living with HIV rather than dying from it is a challenge which cannot be overestimated. This chapter explores HIV infection in infants, children and adolescents, focusing on the family perspective.

Although most accounts of 'paediatric' infection quote vertical transmission as the major source of infection, this is often because other sources are generally overlooked in such analyses, or because the systematic tracking of HIV infection in pregnant women allows for close follow-up of vertically exposed children. Figure 3.1 shows the data for Europe, by way of example, which clearly sets out the differences. In Europe the majority of children (those aged under 13 years) with HIV infection ($n=6,693$ by end 1996) acquired this through horizontal transmission via microtransfusions or contaminated instruments. The majority of such children are based in Romania ($n=3,781$ by end 1996) with another pocket of infection in Russia. This group is followed by children in southern European countries most often associated, directly or indirectly, with injecting drug use. Most accounts of children in Europe, however, set the former larger group aside, and concentrate on those infected through mother-to-child transmission ($n=2,635$). Paediatric infection in Africa is generally associated with heterosexual transmission. In the United States the patterns resemble Europe, with a predominance of children in drug-using, ethnic or impoverished backgrounds. In the early years of the epidemic many paediatric infections were associated with the receipt of blood or blood products (Simonds and Oxtoby, 1995), but in later years the majority of cases are reported in association with mother-to-child transmission, occasionally with attribution to other routes such as sexual, contaminated needles or organ donation.

One of the difficulties in gathering accurate information on children relates to the different definitions of 'child'. European data on children usually uses 13 years as a cut-off point. Yet there are many who would argue that adolescents should be served under this remit. By the end of 1996, a total of 8,100 children under 19 years of age had developed AIDS in Europe. At the same time the numbers of children who are orphaned to AIDS is actually

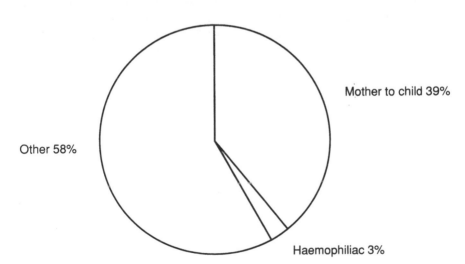

Figure 3.1 *Cumulative totals of cases in children (under 13) in 19 EU countries by September 1996.*

greater than the number of new infections recorded. Global estimates of HIV infection in children shows a growing trend, with over 6 million children infected or affected.

The European collaborative study (European Collaborative Study, 1990, 1994, 1996) has provided the most comprehensive long-term prospective study of mother–infant HIV infection and has shown that vertical transmission in this group has been as low as 12.9% in the early 1990s, but in reports for 1996 it is currently moving upwards slightly to rates approaching 16%. This is accounted for by the growing numbers of women entering the cohort whose risk for HIV is associated with pattern II country origins. Pattern II countries are those described by the World Health Organization where HIV is generally associated with heterosexual spread; it is the predominant mode of HIV infection. Pattern II countries occur in sub-Saharan Africa and the Caribbean. In developing countries generally, sub-Saharan Africa and South America specifically, vertical transmission rates are much higher, closer to 30%. Reported rates for the United States are generally higher than for Europe, but in the most recent years they have shown a dramatic decrease, accounted for by the introduction of AZT (zidovudine) therapy during pregnancy. This decrease is reported in a wide range of studies where the therapy is introduced (Sherr, 1997). Davis *et al.* (1995) calculated the incidence of vertically acquired HIV in children born between 1988 and 1993 and noted that approximately 14,920 infants were born in the United States with HIV between 1978 and 1993. Of these about 12,240 were living at the beginning of 1994, with 26% being under 2 years of age, 35% aged 2–4 and 39% older than 5 years.

Older children and adolescents with HIV are usually infected via earlier transfusion-associated transmission, especially children doubly affected by haemophilia. Others are infected through sexual transmission, sexual abuse and injecting drugs. The data on these groups of children is limited and difficult to combine into a comprehensive body of knowledge on children. There are relatively few studies exploring sexual abuse and HIV infection in children. However, as this is primarily a sexually transmitted disease, it is vital that thorough studies continue and workers understand the mental health implications of sexual abuse, and their enormity when compounded by HIV transmission (Sherr, 1997). Gellert *et al.* (1993) noted that the frequency of HIV transmission due to sexual abuse was increasing and they describe the sensitivity needed when approaching HIV testing in these situations.

The extent of the problem in adolescents is poorly understood with piecemeal documentation. D'Angelo (1994) reports that in the United States as of 30 June 1993, 913 cases of AIDS among adolescents aged 13–19 years had been reported to the Centre for Disease Control (CDC). Kaplan and Schonberg (1994) reported that adolescents comprised only 1% of the total number of individuals reported with AIDS in the United States. Forsyth (1995) reports that 0.2% of American students were HIV positive and 1 in every 278 job corps applicants were HIV positive. One out of every 244 adolescent health clinic attenders tested HIV positive in a Washington study in

1987, increasing fivefold in a five-year follow-up, revealing a rate of 1 in 52 (D'Angelo, 1994). A Medline search identified 220 studies on AIDS and adolescents over 1994–95 (Sherr, 1997). Yet the majority focused on adolescent knowledge, attitudes, behaviours or prevention efforts, and only five examined adolescents with HIV infection or living in a home with others (siblings or parents) who were HIV positive or who had died from an AIDS-related illness (Sherr, 1997).

Vertical Transmission

A range of studies have been set up to explore the relative risks of infant infection according to maternal or birth variables, including time of infection, disease state, treatment and handling. The majority of children born to HIV positive mothers are not themselves infected. Thorough tracking of vertical transmission rates reveals a variation according to geographical distribution, and this may reflect other variables such as virus strain, background medical factors, length of exposure to the virus or socio-economic and drug use issues.

The advent of interventions, notably antiretroviral drugs (Connor *et al.*, 1994), has had a dramatic impact on reducing vertical transmission rates, but the effects of such protocols on the otherwise uninfected infant and the problems for maternal disease management, which may be in conflict with the protocols of combination therapy, have yet to be accurately monitored (Minkoff and Augenbraun, 1997). Attention to pregnancy handling and care has been completely dominated by treatment issues, with scant attention to emotional or mental health needs of this client group. The comprehensive studies often focus on birth parameters, and maternal variables are often confined to medical parameters after the infant is delivered.

Although associated with a statistically significant reduction in vertical transmission – trial ACTG 076 (Connor *et al.*, 1994) – the decisions on antiretroviral treatments in pregnancy are complex. The need to prevent vertical transmission may be pitted against the care needs and drug indications for pregnant women. There is inadequate research for this group, and clinical circumstances, HIV state and previous drug experience may need to be carefully balanced in the choice of interventions for pregnant women. Indeed, Minkoff and Augenbraun (1997) warns that the 'possibility exists that even as new protocols are documented to have therapeutic advantage pregnancy will remain a clinical backwater in which antiretroviral therapy remains focused solely on the prevention of mother to child transmission'. The considerations need to be carefully balanced. Zidovudine monotherapy is now considered non-optimum care in non-pregnant HIV positive clients. Problems with the 076 protocol that need consideration include the creation of drug resistance which will affect the utility of drug regimens for the mother's own health in the future (and thereby reduce the quality and quantity of subsequent mothering); drug side effects, vaginal tumours, resistance and the unknown long-term effects on infants who otherwise would not have been infected.

What has emerged is the variety of interventions, notably drug treatment, avoidance of breast-feeding and delivery management, which have had profound effects on policy for all pregnant women. Many obstetric units now promote HIV testing with all pregnant women. The identification of all positive pregnant women may be at some psychological cost to all clinic attenders, and may result in an upsurge of resource need. Few studies monitor HIV in fathers, promote HIV discussion in family planning, general practice or termination of pregnancy clinics. Furthermore, the availability of a growing number of interventions to limit vertical transmission may have specific effects on the pregnancy intentions and decision making of HIV positive parents. The behavioural associations with the growth in knowledge of vertical transmission should be continuously monitored.

Diagnosis

In the early years of the epidemic, diagnosis was hampered by the presence of maternal antibody in infant blood. This meant that a period of uncertainty, lasting up to two years, would sometimes follow the birth of a child. In more recent times the advent of sophisticated techniques such as polymerase chain reaction (PCR) tests allows for a more rapid definitive diagnosis of newborns, with increasing accuracy as the infant becomes older (Midani and Rathore, 1997; Nesheim *et al.*, 1997). Their availability is now widespread but not universal. Some parents choose not to know the status of their children, while others find the disclosure of diagnosis a challenging task. Melvin and Sherr (1995) studied a consecutive cohort of London HIV positive children and noted that only 7% knew of their HIV status. Even when children know of their status, secrecy often abounds, along with sibling ignorance, wider family ignorance and ignorance of full detail.

Treatments

Most treatment studies have focused on medical treatment of infection, rather than behavioural or management regimes and allied coping and adjustment. From early studies (Belman, Diamond and Dickson, 1988; Belman, 1989, 1992) it was noted that children with gross brain pathology responded positively to AZT administration, which was correlated with reversal of developmental delay symptomatology. Prophylactic treatments avoid both illness episodes, allied psychological harm and incidents of associated hospitalization. However, there is a cost to treatment, including side effects, compliance, negative behaviours surrounding medication administration and unknown long-term effects of medication on functioning. In adults the use of combination therapies has given considerable hope for a reduction in viral load and allied long-term survival. These treatments in children are only now receiving attention, and their long-term implications will need careful monitoring. Early reports show similar advantages for paediatric populations (Englund *et al.*, 1997; Luzuriaga *et al.*, 1997). Yet many countries do not license combination drugs for children; they are available on a named basis only. Some of the regimens associated with combination therapy (timing, fasting, eating, etc.) may be particularly difficult for children. Much research and evaluation is still needed for this population.

Symptom alleviation may well be associated with increased ability to maximize psychological and developmental potential. For example, Hirschfeld *et al.* (1996) noted that 59% of a group of HIV positive children ($n=61$) reported pain as a component of their illness that impacted on their lives. Pain management may thus need to be a component in intervention. There are relatively few interventions for children documented in the literature. The majority of studies focus on the family input. Ideally HIV should be viewed within the family system, and interventions which enhance family adaptation and coping are the most often reported. These studies focus on secrecy (Mok, 1991; Mok and Cooper, 1997; Melvin and Sherr, 1995), stigma (Wiener *et al.*, 1994) and the safety nets provided by families (Ankrah, 1993).

Illness Progression

Children who are HIV positive as a result of vertical transmission seem to fall into two broad categories in terms of illness progression. The first group. includes those who become ill with opportunistic infections early in life, generally around the third month and usually before the first year. This group of children have a poor prognosis. The second group of children are those who remain relatively well. These children may have an oscillating disease course, and many survive within ongoing cohort studies. Children born to women with AIDS are more likely to become infected than those born to HIV positive mothers with no AIDS diagnosis (Abrams *et al.*, 1995). Prematurity in the infant is associated with shorter survival in positive infants (Abrams *et al.*, 1995).

Most research in this area consists of studies on children followed up after maternal exposure. However, there are several studies on children presenting at clinics, and source of infection is rarely controlled for in this cohort. Some of the follow-up reports on children with haemophilia are a notable exception. It is also difficult to make any definitive comments on these different groups until the literature base allows for comparisons.

Evans *et al.* (1997) reported on all ($n=302$) vertically acquired HIV infection in the British Paediatric Association surveillance study. By 1995 over half the children had developed an AIDS indicator disease. Comparisons between these children under 5 years and the general population showed a 2,500 times greater prevalence of non-Hodgkin's lymphoma. Blanche *et al.* (1997) reported on 392 infected children enrolled in two European prospective studies of infants born to HIV positive mothers. They note that the majority of children have experienced either minor or moderately severe illness by the age of 4. Based on this data they note that the risk of death by age 1 year is 20% with a rate of 4.7% per year thereafter. By 6 years of age they report a mortality rate of 26%. Children who survived to the age of 6 were relatively well with two-thirds having only minor symptoms. The European Collaborative Study (ECS) suggests that around one-quarter of children with HIV develop AIDS-defining illnesses before their first birthdays, and by age 4 some 40% of children will have developed AIDS (European Collaborative Study, 1996, 1994). Ramafedi and Lauer (1995) described survival trends in 117 HIV positive adolescents (non-haemophiliacs) and noted that 14% had died of AIDS-related conditions. Survival for this group from diagnosis of HIV was 3 years. Cumulative survival for the cohort at 8 years after diagnosis was 52%. In the face of new treatments, survival issues may present a variety of challenges. Adolescents who anticipated a future of death and illness may respond well to the new combination therapies, and extended survival may require a readjustment plus a need to address a wide range of issues for this group.

Survival

Survival is associated negatively with early onset. Mean survival times from diagnosis to death are shorter in children than adults. Prophylactic interventions and disease management have extended survival times and helped with opportunistic infection avoidance. Extended survival brings with it a host of other problems, often associated with development in the face of life-threatening illnesses, hospitalization, parental illness or multiple bereavement. The developing child may experience virus-associated negative effects, and they are also documented.

Neurological Problems: Cognitive Impairment

Neurological problems are frequently monitored and reported in these children, with findings of developmental delay, neurological symptoms, various learning and cognitive problems, and sometimes specific learning difficulties as they grow older. Armstrong, Seidel and Swales (1993) predict that HIV infection will become the primary infectious cause of perinatally acquired developmental disabilities in the United States. However, other children are recorded as functioning within normal parameters. One should always remember that all vertically infected children are living in a household where the mother, and maybe other family members, are similarly infected.

As early as the late 1980s and early 1990s, central nervous system (CNS) involvement has been noted in children with HIV (Belman, Diamond and Dickson, 1988). Children with HIV are often noted to have developmental delay, loss of milestones, cognitive deficits, language problems and learning difficulties. Burns (1992) noted that 90% of children showed neurologic abnormalities at autopsy. However, it is difficult to specify the relationship between neurological abnormalities and functioning abnormalities, let alone to differentiate between HIV-caused pathogenesis or treatment-related findings. Scarmato *et al.* (1996) noted differential patterns of brain atrophy in pediatric AIDS encephalopathy. Brouwers *et al.* (1995) studied CT (computer tomography) brain scan abnormalities in 87 children and rated abnormalities with intelligence test and social emotional behaviour ratings. Calcifications were associated with greater delays in neurocognitive development.

Comparisons between adults and children in Europe reveal that significantly more children are diagnosed with neurological impairment as their first AIDS-defining diagnosis. This can be clearly seen even when compared with adolescents. An analysis of the European data reveals that by March 1996, 7,269 children had been diagnosed with AIDS: 6,202 in the 1–12 age group and 1,067 in the 13–19 age group. The European Data Centre records neurological AIDS diagnosis for the first four diagnoses. The figures are set out in Table 3.1.

Table 3.1 may reflect an overinclusion of neurological criteria that are not of the same nature as the conditions commonly recorded in adults and described as AIDS dementia complex. The total percentage of neuropsychological diagnoses across the first four reported diagnostic categories in the younger age group is 2.32% (*n*=144) of the whole sample (*n*=6,202), considerably higher than 0.56% (*n*=6) in the older group (*n*=1,067). Any developmental delay or loss of milestone is usually recorded as neurological impairment, and this may be an overdiagnosed condition covering a wide variety of symptoms in children with HIV disease. Clear refining of the

Table 3.1 *Proportion of neuropsychological diagnostic categories of AIDS indicator diseases for children with AIDS in Europe (up to March 1996)*[a]

Age group	*N*	Diagnosis 1[b]		Diagnosis 2[b]		Diagnosis 3[b]		Diagnosis 4[b]	
		n	%	*n*	%	*n*	%	*n*	%
1–12 year olds	6,202	76	1.2	38	0.6	21	0.3	9	0.2
13–19 year olds	1,067	0	0	2	0.2	3	0.3	1	0.1

[a] Data acknowledged with thanks from the Paris Centre database.
[b] Diagnoses refer to the first four presenting diagnoses recorded for each child with AIDS.

concept is urgently needed for this group. O'Hara (1995) describes primary neurological abnormalities and secondary neurological complications that result from immunodeficiency and produce opportunistic infections of the CNS.

Methodological Problems with Neurological Investigations

The true incidence, range and content of childhood neurological problems associated with HIV is unclear; some writers claim it is underreported (Turner *et al.*, 1995) whereas others show a widely divergent range depending on the place where studies are carried out. In the United States, the reported rates are as high as 90% compared to European children, where recorded rates are closer to 20–30% (Msellati *et al.*, 1993; European Collaborative Study, 1996). There are a wide range of methodological problems associated with the description and diagnosis of neurological problems in children with HIV. Some cohort studies are drawn from clinic populations, which disproportionately include those with impairment who have been diagnosed with HIV disease on the appearance of neurological symptoms. The more sophisticated studies compare HIV positive children born to HIV positive mothers and use either HIV negative children born to positive mothers, or HIV negative siblings. They are more reliable because they account for the potential developmental impact of an ill, dying or absent mother and developmental disruption of family illness and disease management. Other methodological problems surround some of the major risks associated with maternal infection in the first place. For example, in Europe (Spain, France, Italy and Portugal specifically) maternal drug use is a major route of HIV infection and may itself affect development. Other categories of maternal infection, such as migration from areas of high prevalence, may also affect cognitive development in young children if such parents are ill, migrants, isolated from wider family, economically disadvantaged and having a home (and first) language which differs from the test centre and the test items. The range of test inventories is problematic in itself, but often involves translation and translocation, hence validity and accurate normative data are questionable. The Bayley scales of infant development are often used (Nozyce *et al.*, 1994a,b).

Few studies have designs which are sufficiently sophisticated to control for problems such as low birthweight and premature delivery, factors commonly associated with HIV positive children and also well noted in the literature as possible contributors to developmental differences. Among some cohorts, there are multiple problems and it is difficult to differentiate them and the extent to which they contribute to findings. Examples include children with HIV and haemophilia (Hilgartner *et al.*, 1993) or parental drug use. Some studies use retrospective analysis (Mok *et al.*, 1996) and very few report that the assessors are blind to the serostatus of the child.

Development

Developmental delay has been discussed in relation to HIV positive children from the earliest cases. Blanche *et al.* (1994), working in Paris, has noted that there is a relationship between maternal illness at birth and CNS involvement in subsequently infected children. Despite concerns about widespread delay, and early calls for planning special education, later studies have shown the picture to be more complex. Whitt *et al.* (1993) examined children with haemophilia and integrated blind examinations into the design where six domains for neuropsychological functioning were measured. They found no differences between groups of similar age, race and socio-economic status according to HIV status. Subtle deficits were noted when the data was compared to age norms. They concluded that it was difficult to attribute early subtle neuropsychological deficits to this group of haemophilic children to CNS effects of HIV. Nozyce *et al.* (1994a,b) studied 181 children with a range of standardised inventories. Children who were HIV positive ($n=21$) were compared with those born to HIV positive mothers who were uninfected ($n=65$) and those born to HIV negative mothers, matched on sociodemographic variables ($n=95$). They reported that children with AIDS, i.e. those with opportunistic infections, showed cognitive impairment whereas those who were HIV positive and well showed developmental profiles not dissimilar from control children. The association between developmental problems and neurological problems is also unclear. Msellati *et al.* (1993) noted that children with HIV disease often have abnormal neurological examination outcomes, and children as young as 12 or 18 months showed motor problems. Aylward *et al.* (1992) looked at young infants (5.5 to 24 months) comparing seronegatives ($n=45$) seropositives ($n=12$) and seroreverters ($n=39$) and found significant group differences on the mental development index and psychomotor development index of the Bayley scales. Seropositive infants scored lower than the other groups.

A number of small-scale studies have been reported which show the progress on a range of standardized measures over time. For example, Tardieu *et al.* (1995) studied a small number of HIV positive children ($n=33$) and found that over one-third achieved at normal school age rates. Problems for HIV positive children were more discrete and were found to be associated with specific tasks such as visuospatial and language areas. Papola, Alvarez and Cohen (1994) looked at school age children with HIV; they noted cognitive and learning deficits yet reported that children were functioning better than originally predicted. Hilgartner *et al.* (1993) studied children and adolescents infected with both haemophilia and HIV and showed that on a battery of neuropsychological tests the HIV positive children were 50% more likely to score on standard deviation below expected levels in one-third of the areas. However, the difference was not significant, and these results should be interpreted with caution. The small sample size should be considered as well as the wide age range in this study (6 to 19 years). And the effects of additional chronic illness must be taken into account as it can directly affect learning by simple factors such as school absence. It is also unclear what the differences are on a developing cognitive system in the case of younger children, and an older child. Levenson *et al.* (1992) concluded that cognitive functioning in their sample of HIV positive children was below average, with particular problems in memory tests and verbal scores. Language problems were noted and these may have interacted with other areas given that many test directions are language dependent.

Language problems have been found by a number of workers, but not identified as problematic for others. For example, Havens *et al.* (1993) noted no differences in language functioning for HIV positive children compared to HIV negative controls, but confirmed memory and reasoning disparities. Nozyce *et al.* (1994b) noted that impairments were mostly observed in children who subsequently developed opportunistic infections by the age of 24 months. Moss *et al.* (1996) studied expressive behaviours in 83 HIV-infected children in the United States, comparing children with encephalopathic or non-encephalopathic classifications. The non-encephalopathic group displayed higher activity levels, had superior motor verbal skills and exhibited greater social skills and emotional responsiveness. Wolters *et al.* (1995) examined the effects on receptive and expressive language development and compared this to CT brain scan abnormalities in 36 children with symptomatic HIV infection along with 20 uninfected siblings. Expressive language was more impaired than receptive language for all children. Those with encephalopthy had lower scores whereas siblings showed no such discrepancy and scored higher than the infected children. CT scan abnormalities were related to lowered expressive and receptive language functioning, particularly in the group with encephalopathy. These authors believe the findings can be explained directly by HIV-related CNS effects. Lobato *et al.* (1995) reported on the incidence, characteristics and survival of children with perinatally acquired HIV and encephalopathy generated from a sample of 1,811 children where 178 (23%) were diagnosed with enceophalopathy out of 766 children with AIDS diagnoses. The condition resulted in more hospitalizations and a similar survival pattern to children with PCP, which was as short as 22 months.

Mother and Family Effects

Clearly the data focuses on children with HIV infection, but it is also important to track any developmental delay in children cared for by an HIV positive mother, or in uninfected children born to an HIV positive mother. Continuous exposure to problems in family life may contribute to developmental problems for all children. Mok *et al.* (1996) examined routine child health information for 459 children to explore the impact of HIV infection and drug use during pregnancy. No differences were noted on developmental progress, but medical consultations in the first 18 months of life did vary with maternal drug use associated with lower consulting rates. It is unclear, however, whether consulting rates are an index of development. Indeed, they may simply be a surrogate marker for illness, given that HIV positive mothers may be more likely to consult for their own condition, and bring their child with them. But it was notable that, despite early intact families, by 10 months only 81% of the children born to HIV-infected drug-using women lived with a biological parent. Table 3.2 summarizes the studies to date.

Behaviour Problems

Early reports from the United States described behaviour problems in HIV positive children. However, it was unclear whether they were associated with infection; the background factors in the family which predisposed to infection, particularly drug use but also separations, constant disruptions, bereavement or loss; medication side effects; illness effects; or a combination of everything. Early studies tend to be descriptive and uncontrolled for these variables. They can thus point out the future needs for this client group but cannot begin to unravel causative factors, contributory factors or theoretical explanations. In the absence of theoretical explanations, prevention becomes problematic and rarely discussed. Subsequent studies report varied findings, depending on approach, country of study and measurement parameters. Havens *et al.* (1994) noted behavioural problems in HIV positive children, but associated them with drug use and noted that negative children also exposed to maternal drugs had similar rates of behavioural problems. In African studies the impact of the family disruption, orphanhood and maternal illness have all shown that behavioural sequelae are expected concomitants of HIV infection. These studies showed HIV positivity as a compounding factor rather than a causal factor.

The true aetiology of behavioural problems may not be discernible. If the virus does cross the blood–brain barrier and affect children neurologically at times of development, ramifications may be expected. However, it seems impossible and perhaps undesirable to attempt to isolate pure virus implications on development without understanding the dramatic psychological impact of this disease on childhood development, behaviour and environment. It would be impossible to disentangle the various factors, let alone quantify them. Suffice it to say that studies have come up with disparate findings but all specify the theme of potential behavioural problems, and care packages need to accommodate the harsh circumstances experienced by children in families where HIV has permeated.

Emotional and Psychological Considerations

Mental health burdens are wide-ranging and extend beyond the HIV positive child to all those living in an HIV-affected family. The multiple nature of the

Table 3.2 *Summary of studies reporting on development in children with HIV infection*

Study	N	Place	Findings
Bouvin *et al.* (1995)	14 HIV+ 20 reverters 16 control	Zaire	Denver developmental screening tests used. Developmental delay recorded. Motor and visual spatial deficits noted, even in asymptomatic children. Maternal infection undermines cognitive development in uninfected children.
Chase *et al.* (1995)	24 HIV+ 27 reverters	USA	Bayley scales. Motor development in the infected group was delayed. Mental development comparable. HIV infection associated with delay in mental development. Early motor delay common but variability noted.
Msellati *et al.* (1993)	436 children 218 mum HIV+[a] 218 mum HIV−	Rwanda	Motor problems for 31% of 1-year-olds, 40% of 1.5-year-olds. Only 1 severe encephalopathy in 50 HIV+ children. Proportion of abnormal neurological examinations always higher than uninfected children. Much of the developmental delay was due to lower motor scores. Delay related to stage of AIDS.
Nozyce (1994a,b)	21 HIV+ 65 reverters 95 HIV−	USA	HIV+ symptomatic children significantly lower. HIV+ well children similar to controls. Uninfected and asymptomatic children have relatively normal neurodevelopment.
Tardieu *et al.* (1995)			29% show affective disorders.
Hittleman, Nelson and Shah (1993)		USA	Attention problems in 53% HIV+ children.
Havens *et al.* (1994)			Disruptive behaviours noted, associated with maternal drug use.
Hooper *et al.* (1993)		USA	No differences (haemophiliac children).

Table 3.2 *Continued*

Study	N	Place	Findings
Mellins and Ehrhardt (1994)	25 families	USA	Children particularly vulnerable to separation and loss; siblings reported anger and burden from caregiving tasks.
Hilgartner *et al.* (1993)	n = 333 62% HIV+ 38% HIV−	USA	HIV+ are three times as likely to show height decline, twice as likely to show delays in sexual maturation, and 50% more likely to show scores one standard deviation below expected levels in three of nine functional areas.
Aylward *et al.* (1992)	n = 96 12 HIV+ 39 reverters 45 HIV−	USA	Bayley scales on infants aged 5.5 to 24 months. Significant differences on mental development index and psychomotor development index (positive children lower than negative or reverters).
McKinney and Robertson (1993)	n = 170 62 HIV+ 10 HIV−	USA	HIV-infected children have significantly smaller weight for age, and length for age.
Piazza *et al.* (1995)	n = 138 58 HIV+ 80 reverted	Italy	Incidence of central nervous system involvement was 36% for symptomatic HIV. Development deficit and psychological problems prevalent in infected and uninfected children without group differences.
Burns (1992)		USA	Some 90% of paediatric AIDS autopsies revealed abnormalities.
Depas *et al.* (1995)	8	France	Hypometabolism and subcortical hypermetabolism were found in three children with severe neurological signs. Functional abnormalities precede clinical symptoms.
Gay *et al.* (1995)	n = 126 128 HIV+ 98 HIV−	USA	Mean mental and motor scores of HIV+ infants significantly lower than HIV− controls. Difference increased over time. Yet one-third of the infected infants exhibited relatively normal cognitive development and one-half demonstrated relatively normal motor development.

Table 3.2 *Continued*

Study	N	Place	Findings
Whitt *et al.* (1993)	n=63 25 HIV+ 38 HIV−	USA[b]	Six domains of functioning assessed blind. No differences in groups of similar age, race and socio-economic status defined by HIV status. High incidence of subtle deficits revealed when compared to age norms.
Bell *et al.* (1997)	n=153 76 HIV+ 77 HIV−	Côte d'Ivoire	Low prevalence of HIV encephalitis – explained by the comparatively early death in HIV-infected children in Africa compared to Western children.

[a] Of the children born to HIV+ mothers, 50 were HIV+ themselves.
[b] People with haemophilia.

burdens, and their ramifications on all members of the family may lead to a complex web of interrelated emotional trauma without much precedent in the literature. The crucial questions of understanding, predicting and service provision should not be overlooked if prevention of strain or amelioration of burden is to be incorporated into care plans. In summarizing the areas considered above, it is helpful to look separately at infected children, their parents, their siblings and others.

Infected Children

Cohen (1994) reviewed studies to understand the impact and long-term effects on families. These studies point out the unique constellation of factors which may render HIV/AIDS unparalleled in its multiple burdening. They also explore the need to focus positively, whereas many studies focus negatively and overlook concepts such as resilience. Forsyth *et al.* (1996) noted that children in families with HIV infection were more withdrawn, and HIV positive children had more attention-related problems. Havens *et al.* (1994) describe behaviour problems but associate this with drug use, either instead of HIV or as well as HIV. Behaviour problems are often the first ramification of any uncertainty, disruption, fear, anxiety or concern experienced by the child.

Grief and bereavement are aspects of mental health and development that simply cannot be overlooked in this group of children. From the moment that fatal illness is diagnosed in a family, bereavement and loss become an issue for all children, both positive and negative. Indeed, studies that simply track development and mental health adjustment in HIV positive children are limited, as all children affected by HIV may have long-term consequences.

Multiple family infection is the norm, and dual challenge with other conditions is common. Refugee and migrant issues also abound among affected families (Melvin and Sherr, 1995).

Parents

McShane, Bumbalo and Patsdaughter (1994) described the range of psychological distress measured in family members living with someone who has HIV/AIDS in a sample of 133 persons from 80 families, including parents ($n=47$) siblings ($n=53$) and adult family members ($n=33$). They found that parents, siblings and people living with AIDS revealed higher overall distress levels and higher symptoms on the brief symptom inventory compared to norms. Forsyth *et al.* (1996) assessed mental health functioning of children with HIV positive mothers and compared this to matched children of HIV negative mothers in the United States. Items used included the child behaviour checklist, adapted childhood anxiety scales and depression inventories. Children of HIV positive mothers were significantly more withdrawn, reported more attention-related problems and higher rates of depression than control children. Total behaviour checklist scores and anxiety, however, did not differ.

Mellins and Ehrhardt (1994) studied stress and coping in families affected with HIV by interviewing all family members in a cohort of 25 affected families. They noted that the majority of caregivers were single mothers who experienced disproportionate isolation, caregiving responsibilities, lack of resources and support. Separation and loss were particular problems for all children (negative and positive). They also point out the anger and burdensome caregiving tasks shouldered by negative siblings. Although they did monitor them, they predicted that coping resources would be stretched over time, and they concluded that support or early intervention would be helpful. Roth *et al.* (1994) go further; they describe how additional stresses are a burden to these families. There may be stigma, poverty, children who often experience disrupted nurturing, constant separations and unpredictable environments filled with change, economic hardship and disruptions in routine.

Throughout the literature there is a call for early testing. This has profound implications for all children who are exposed to HIV testing, the trauma around the decision to test, the consideration of HIV as a possible diagnosis in the case of an ill child, and the subsequent management of mental health and emotional trauma in the event of a positive test result.

Siblings

Siblings are often the silent group of children deeply affected by this epidemic, but rarely studied, other than in the capacity of control groups. Yet they are directly affected by infection in the family. The nature of infection is such that it is not uncommon for multiple family infection. The affected child carries the burden of disrupted family, loss and separation, secrecy, disrupted parenting, disproportionate attention to the ill child and a number of associated hardships that are the inevitable companions of this infection. They include poverty, financial hardship, economic burden and exclusion. Melvin and Sherr (1995) found that siblings were invariably kept in ignorance of family infection. They often have to assume caretaking responsibility and in many areas become the primary carer of ill siblings if parental death occurs.

The long-term damage on such children has simply not been documented, although the growing burden of orphans is now being catalogued in the literature (Foster *et al.*, 1995). The growing orphan problem will create wide-ranging problems. Kamali *et al.* (1996) studied a rural population in Uganda where seroprevalence of HIV was 8% among adults and found that over 10% of children under the age of 15 had lost one or both parents. Paternal loss was more common than maternal loss (6.3% compared to 2.8%). Continued loss was monitored in this cohort at a rate of 43% over three years. It was notable that school attendance was affected by orphanhood, a factor which may compound developmental achievements.

Foster *et al.* (1995) tracked the number of orphans in 570 households in Zimbabwe and noted that by 1992 some 18.3% included orphans mostly under 15 years of age. Much of the care was located in the extended families, which suffered from strains but did not discriminate or exploit the orphaned children. Of note in this study was the emergence of sibling-headed orphaned families. Studies in different centres show different priorities. Levine (1995) listed some of the unmet needs for orphaned US children, particularly in relation to mental health services. These workers estimated that by the end of 1995 maternal death caused by HIV/AIDS would have orphaned 24,600 children and 21,000 adolescents in the United States. By the end of 1991 some 13% of US children and 9% of adolescents whose mothers had died of all causes, had deaths which were associated with AIDS.

Schable *et al.* (1995) studied 541 HIV positive women in ten US centres and noted that 88% had living children, 49% with more than one child. Caretaking patterns were mixed; most often noted was the scenario of a single mother (46%); grandparents existed in 16% of cases and mother and father in only 15%. Ryder *et al.* (1994) studied the psychosocial and economic impact on orphaned children over a four-year period in Kinshasa. A total of 1,072 children were studied, and orphaned children were (1) compared with a group living with an HIV positive mother who was alive and (2) compared with an HIV negative mother. Orphan rates were 8.2 per 100 HIV seropositive women years of follow-up. The availability of a caring extended family buffeted these growing children against adverse health and socio-economic effects.

Others

There are a number of others who are affected within families, including grandparents, carers and those who provide all forms of support for families and children. A true family perspective is really needed to catalogue the web of effects. Grandparents, for example, may be called upon to provide childcare. This may be for well or sick children. And it may be in the face of their own child's illness or death. The needs of grandparents who may be frail and reliant on the next generation will be totally overlooked if they are relied on to be providers rather than receivers of care. Aunts, uncles, cousins and friends are all inevitably drawn in. In some cultures the extended family is the core of support networks. These are often stretched to their limits, or even to breaking point in some centres (Ankrah, 1993). Carers, from voluntary sector to health care service, are also affected and very few studies have documented their needs, their burdens or the interventions which successfuly alleviate them.

Conclusion

The mental health effects of HIV on children and families is profound. The causes are either directly related to the virus and associated illness, or indirectly related to the complex circumstances invariably assocated with HIV disease. The advent of treatments and interventions to prevent vertical transmission may shift the balance so that mental health needs finally emerge as overwhelming. The predominant focus on drugs and treatments has often diverted attention from the profound and often multiple burden of HIV on the emotional well-being of the family. Provision has often also lagged behind. There are few areas of literature which can provide a precedent or a background to understand HIV. Any generalizations must indicate the need to sustain quality of family life and continuity of care as well as the need to support all family members before, during and after the many crises associated with the course of HIV disease. Any failure to provide fully will ramify through the generations.

Acknowledgements

I acknowledge the European study on ante-natal HIV testing policy and procedure, jointly held with Professor C. Hudson; Women and AIDS Healthy Alliance study in collaboration with Dr M. Johnston, Dr J. Elford, Ms R. Miller and Ms H. Wells, and the European Commission study on legal services for discrimination in AIDS and HIV cases, with Professor Avrom Sherr. Specific thanks are extended to the Paris Centre, Dr F. Hammers and Dr A. Downs within the framework of the EC Multinational

Scenario Analysis, who provided access to the European data set for analysis of neurological diagnosis among children in Europe. This chapter is dedicated to Neil O'May.

References

ABRAMS, E., MATHESON, P., THOMAS, P., THEA, D., KRASINKSKI, K. and LAMBERT, G. (1995) 'Neonatal predictors of infection status and early death among 332 infants at risk of HIV 1 infection monitored prospectively from birth', *Pediatrics*, **96**, 3, pp. 451–58.

ANKRAH, E.M. (1993) 'The impact of HIV/AIDS on the family and other significant relationships – the African clan revisited', *AIDS Care*, **5**, 1, pp. 5–23.

ARMSTRONG, F., SEIDEL, J. and SWALES, T. (1993) 'Pediatric HIV infection: a neuropsychological and educational challenge', *Journal of Learning Disabilities*, **26**, 2, pp. 92–103.

AYLWARD, E., BUTZ, A., HUTTON, N., JOYNER, M. and VOGELHUT, J. (1992) 'Cognitive and motor development in infants at risk for HIV', *American Journal of Diseases in Children*, **146**, 2, pp. 218–22.

BELL, J., LOWRIE, S., KOFFI, K., HONDE, M., ANDOH, J., DE COCK, K. and LUCAS, S. (1997) 'The neuropathology of HIV infected African children in Abidjan, Cote d'Ivoire', *Journal of Neuropathology and Experimental Neurology*, **56**, 6, pp. 686–92.

BELMAN, A. (1989) 'Neurological aspects of children with HIV', paper presented at the WHO Mothers and Babies Conference, Paris.

BELMAN, A. (1992) 'AIDS and the child's CNS', *Pediatric Clinics of North America*, **39**, 4, pp. 691–714.

BELMAN, A., DIAMOND, G. and DICKSON, D. (1988) 'Pediatric acquired immunodeficiency syndrome – neurological syndromes', *Journal of Diseases in Children*, **142**, pp. 29–35.

BLANCHE, S., MAYAUX, M., ROUZIOUX, C., TEGLAS, J., FIRTION, G., MONPOUX, F., CIRARU VIGNERON, N., MEIER, F., TRICOIRE, F., COURPOTIN, C., VILMER, E., GRISCELLI, C. and DELFRAISSY, J. (1994) 'Relation of the course of HIV infection in children to the severity of the disease in their mothers at delivery', *New England Journal of Medicine*, **330**, 5, pp. 308–12.

BLANCHE, S., NEWELL, M.L., MAYAUX, M.-J., DUNN, D., TEGLAS, J., ROUZIOUX, C. and PECKHAM, C. (1997) 'Morbidity and mortality in European children vertically infected by HIV-1', *Journal of Acquired Immune Deficiency Syndrome and Human Retrovirology*, **14**, 5, pp. 442–50.

BOUVIN, M., GREEN, S., DAVIES, A., GIORDANI, B., MOKILI, J. and CUTTING, W. (1995) 'A preliminary evaluation of the cognitive and motor effects of pediatric HIV infection in Zairian children', *Health Psychology*, **14**, 1, pp. 13–21.

Brouwers, P., DeCarli, C., Civitello, L., Moss, H., Wolters, P. and Pizzo, P. (1995) 'Correlation between computed tomographic brain scan abnormalities and neuropsychological function in children with symptomatic HIV disease', *Archives of Neurology*, **52**, 1, pp. 39–44.

Burns, D. (1992) 'The neuropathology of pediatric AIDS', *Journal of Child Neurology*, **7**, 4, pp. 332–46.

Chase, C., Vibbert, M., Pelton, S., Coulter, D. and Cabral, H. (1995) 'Early neurodevelopmental growth in children with vertically transmitted HIV infection', *Archives of Pediatric and Adolescent Medicine*, **149**, 8, pp. 850–55.

Cohen, F. (1994) 'Research on families and pediatric HIV disease: a review and needed directions', *Journal of Developmental and Behavioral Pediatrics*, **15**, 3, pp. s34–42.

Connor, E., Sperling, R., Gelber, R., Kiseley, P., Scott, G.O. and Sullivan, M. (1994) 'Reduction of maternal infant transmission of HIV type 1 with zidovudine treatment', *New England Journal of Medicine*, **331**, pp. 1173–80.

D'Angelo, L. (1994) 'HIV infection and AIDS in adolescents', in Pizzo, P. and Wilfert, C. (eds) *Pediatric AIDS: the challenge of HIV infection in infants, children and adolescents*, 2nd edn, Baltimore MD: Williams and Wilkins.

Davis, S., Byers, R., Lindegren, M., Caldwell, M., Karon, J. and Gwinn, M. (1995) 'Prevalence and incidence of vertically acquired HIV infection in the United States', *JAMA*, **274**, 12, pp. 952–55.

Depas, G., Chiron, C., Tardieu, M., Nuttin, C., Blanche, S., Raynaud, C. and Syrota, A. (1995) 'Functional brain imaging in HIV1 infected children born to seropositive mothers', *Journal of Nuclear Medicine*, **36**, 12, pp. 2169–74.

European Collaborative Study (1990) 'Neurological signs in young children with HIV', *Paediatraic Infectious Diseases Journal*, **9**, pp. 402–6.

European Collaborative Study (1994) 'Natural history of vertically acquired HIV-1 infection', *Pediatrics*, **94**, pp. 815–19.

European Collaborative Study (1996) 'Characteristics of pregnant HIV 1 infected women in Europe', *AIDS Care*, **8**, 1, pp. 33–42.

Englund, J., Baker, C., Raskino, C., McKinney, R., Petrie, B. and Fowler, M. (1997) 'Zidovudine didanosine or both as the initial treatment for symptomatic HIV infected children', *New England Journal of Medicine*, **336**, 24, pp. 1704–12.

Evans, J., Gibb, D., Holland, F., Tookey, P., Pritchard, J. and Ades, A. (1997) 'Malignancies in UK children with HIV infection acquired from mother to child transmission', *Archives of Disease in Childhood*, **76**, 4, pp. 330–33.

Forsyth, B. (1995) 'A pandemic out of control: the epidemiology of AIDS', in Geballe, S.G., Gruendel, J. and Andiman, W. *Forgotten Children of the AIDS Epidemic*, New Haven CT: Yale University Press.

FORSYTH, B., DAMOUR, L., NAGLER, S. and ADNOPOZ, J. (1996) 'The psychological effects of parental HIV infection on uninfected children', *Archives of Pediatric and Adolescent Medicine*, **150**, 10, pp. 1015–20.

FOSTER, G., SHAKESPEARE, R., CHINEMANA, F., JACKSON, H., GREGSON, S., MARANGE, C. and MASHUMBA, S. (1995) 'Orphan prevalence and extended family care in a peri-urban community in Zimbabwe', *AIDS Care*, **7**, 1, pp. 3–19.

GAY, C., ARMSTRONG, F., COHEN, D., LAI, S., HARDY, M., SWALES, T., MORROW, C. and SCOTT, G. (1995) 'The effects of HIV on cognitive and motor development in children born to HIV seropositive women with no reported drug use: birth to 24 months', *Pediatrics*, **96**, 6, pp. 1078–82.

GELLERT, G., BERKOWITZ, C., GELLERT, M. and DURFEE, M. (1993) 'Testing the sexually abused child for the HIV antibody: issues for the social worker', *Social Work*, **38**, 4, pp. 389–94.

HAVENS, J., WHITAKER, A., FELDMAN, J. and EHRHARDT, A. (1994) 'Psychiatric morbidity in school age children with congenital HIV infection', *Developmental and Child Pediatrics*, **15**, 3, pp. s18–25.

HILGARTNER, M., DONFIELD, S., WILLOUGHBY, A., CONTANT, C., EVATT, B., GOMPERTS, E., HOOTS, W., JASON, J., LOVELAND, K. and MCKINLAY, S. (1993) 'Hemophilia growth and development study: design methods and entry data', *American Journal of Pediatric Hematology and Oncology*, **15**, 2, pp. 208–18.

HIRSCHFELD, S., MOSS, H., DRAGISIC, K., SMITH, W. and PIZZO, P. (1996) 'Pain in pediatric HIV infection', *Pediatrics*, **98**, 3, pp. 449–52.

HITTLEMAN, J., NELSON, N. and SHAH, V. (1993) 'Neurodevelopmental disabilities in infants born to HIV infected mothers', *AIDS Reader*, pp. 126–32.

HOOPER, S., WHITT, J., TENNISON, M., BURCHINAL, M., GOLD, S. and HALL, C. (1993) 'Behavioral adaptation to HIV seropositive status in children and adolescents with haemophilia', *American Journal of Diseases in Childhood*, **147**, pp. 541–45.

KAMALI, A., SEELEY, J., NUNN, A., KENGEY, A., KAYONDO, J., RUBERANTWARI, A. and MULDER, D. (1996) 'The orphan problem: experience of a sub-Saharan African rural population in the AIDS epidemic', *AIDS Care*, **8**, 5, pp. 509–15.

KAPLAN, M. and SCHONBERG, S. (1994) 'HIV in adolescents', *Clinical Perinatology*, **21**, pp. 75–84.

LEVENSON, R., MELINS, C., ZAWADZKI, R., KAIRAM, R. and STEIN, Z. (1992) 'Cognitive assessment of HIV exposed children', *American Journal of Diseases in Childhood*, **146**, pp. 1479–83.

LEVINE, C. (1995) 'Orphans of the HIV epidemic: unmet needs in six US cities', *AIDS Care*, **7**, suppl. 1, pp. 57–63.

LOBATO, M., CALDWELL, B., NG, P. and OXTOBY, M. (1995) 'Encephalopathy in children with perinatally acquired HIV infection', *Journal of Pediatrics*, **126**, 5, pp. 710–15.

LUZURIAGA, K., BRYSON, Y., KROGSTAD, P., ROBINSON, J., STECHENBERG, B. and LAMSON, M. (1997) 'Combination treatment with zidovudine, didanosine and nevirapine in infants with HIV-1 infection', *New England Journal of Medicine*, **336**, 9, pp. 1343–49.

MCKINNEY, R. and ROBERTSON, J. (1993) 'Effect of HIV infection on growth of young children', *Journal of Pediatrics*, **123**, 4, pp. 579–82.

MCSHANE, R., BUMBALO, J. and PATSDAUGHTER, C. (1994) 'Psychological distress in family members living with HIV/AIDS', *Archives of Psychiatric Nursing*, **8**, 1, pp. 53–61.

MELLINS, C. and EHRHARDT, A. (1994) 'Families affected by pediatric AIDS: sources of stress and coping', *Journal of Developmental and Behavioural Pediatrics*, **15**, 3, pp. s54–60.

MELVIN, D. and SHERR, L. (1995) 'HIV infection in London children: psychosocial complexity and emotional burden', *Child Care, Health and Development*, **21**, 6, pp. 405–12.

MIDANI, S. and RATHORE, M. (1997) 'PCR testing for early detection of HIV infection in children', *South Medical Journal*, **90**, 3, pp. 294–95.

MINKOFF, H. and AUGENBRAUN, M. (1997) 'Antiretroviral therapy for pregnant women', *American Journal of Obstetrics and Gynecology*, **176**, 2, pp. 478–89.

MOK, J. (1991) 'The medical management of children with HIV disease', in Claxton, R. and Harrison, T. (eds) *Caring for Children with HIV and AIDS*, London: Edward Arnold.

MOK, J. and COOPER, S. (1997) 'The needs of children whose mothers have HIV infection', *Archives of Disease in Childhood*, **77**, 6, pp. 483–87.

MOK, J. and NEWELL, M. (1995) *HIV infection in children – a guide to practical management*, Cambridge: Cambridge University Press.

MOK, J.Y., ROSS, A., RAAB, G., HAMILTON, B., GILKISON, S. and JOHNSTONE, F.D. (1996) 'Maternal HIV and drug use: effect on health and social morbidity', *Archives of Disease in Childhood*, **74**, 3, pp. 210–14.

MOSS, H., WOLTERS, P., BROUWERS, P., HENDRICKS, M. and PIZZO, P. (1996) 'Impairment of expressive behavior in pediatric HIV infected patients with evidence of CNS disease', *Journal of Pediatric Psychology*, **21**, 3, pp. 379–400.

MSELLATI, P., LEPAGE, P., HITIMANA, D., VAN GOETHEM, C., VAN DE PERRE, P. and DABIS, F. (1993) 'Neurodevelopmental testing of children born to HIV type 1 seropositive and seronegative mothers: a prospective cohort study in Kigali Rwanda', *Pediatarics*, **92**, 6, pp. 843–48.

NESHEIM, S., LEE, F., KALISH, M., OU, C., SAWYER, M. and CLARK, S. (1997) 'Diagnosis of perinatal HIV by PCR and p24 antigen detection after immune complex dissocation in an urban community hospital', *Journal of Infectious Diseases*, **175**, 6, pp. 1333–36.

NOZYCE, M., HITTELMAN, J., MUENZ, L., DURAKO, S., FISCHER, M. and WILLOUGHBY, A. (1994a) 'Effect of perinatally acquired HIV infection on neurodevelopment in children during the first two years of life', *Pediatrics*, **94**, 6, pp. 883–91.

NOZYCE, M., HOBERMAN, M., ARPADI, S., WIZNIA, A., LAMBERT, G., DOBROSZYCKI, J., CHANG, A. and ST LOUIS, Y. (1994b) 'A 12 month study of the effects of oral zidovudine on neurodevelopmental functioning in a cohort of vertically HIV infected inner city children', *AIDS*, **8**, pp. 635–39.

O'HARA, M. (1995) 'Care of children with HIV infection', in Kelly, P., Holman, S., Rothenberg, R. and Holzemer, S.P. (eds) *Primary care of women and children with HIV infection*, Boston MA: Jones and Bartlett.

PAPOLA, P., ALVAREZ, M. and COHEN, H. (1994) 'Developmental and service needs of school age children with HIV infection: a descriptive study', *Pediatrics*, **94**, 6, pp. 914–18.

PIAZZA, F., ASTORI, M., MACCABRUNI, A., CASELLI, D., BOSSI, G. and LANZI, G. (1995) 'Neuropsychological development of children born to HIV positive mothers', *Pediatria Medica e Chirugica*, **17**, 4, pp. 331–33.

RAMAFEDI, G. and LAUER, T. (1995) 'Survival trends in adolescents with HIV infection', *Archives of Pediatric and Adolescent Medicine*, **149**, 10, pp. 1093–96.

RYDER, R., KAMENGA, M., NKUSU, M., BATTER, V. and HEYWARD, W. (1994) 'AIDS orphans in Kinshasa, Zaire: incidence and socioeconomic consequences', *AIDS*, **8**, pp. 673–79.

SCARMATO, V., FRANK, Y., ROZENSTEIN, A., LU, D., HYMAN, R. and BAKSHI, S. (1996) 'Central brain atrophy in childhood AIDS enceophalopathy', *AIDS*, **10**, 11, pp. 1227–31.

SCHABLE, B., DIAZ, T., CHU, S. *et al.* (1995) 'Who are the primary caretakers of children born to HIV infected mothers? Results from a mulistate surveillance project', *Pediatrics*, **95**, pp. 511–15.

SHERR, L. (1997) 'Adolescents in our midst', in Sherr, L. (ed.) *AIDS and Adolescents*, Amsterdam: Harwood Academic.

SIMONDS, R. and OXTOBY, M. (1995) 'Epidemiology and natural history of HIV infection in children', in Kelly, P., Holman, S., Rothenberg, R. and Holzemer, S.P. (eds) *Primary care of women and children with HIV infection*, Boston MA: Jones and Bartlett.

TARDIEU, M., MAYAUX, M., SEIBEL, N., FUNCK BRENTANO, I., STRAUB, I., TEGLAS, J. and BLANCHE, S. (1995) 'Cognitive assessment of school age children infected with maternally transmitted HIV type 1', *Journal of Pediatrics*, **126**, pp. 375–79.

TURNER, B., EPPES, S., MCKEE, L., COSLER, L. and MRKON, L. (1995) 'A population based comparison of the clinical course of children and adults with AIDS', *AIDS*, **9**, pp. 65–72.

WHITT, J., HOOPER, S., TENNISON, M., ROBERTSON, W., GOLD, S., BURCHINAL, M., WELLS, R., MCMILLAN, C., WHALEY, R. and COMBEST, J. (1993) 'Neuropsychologic functioning of HIV infected children with haemophilia', *Journal of Pediatrics*, **122**, 1, pp. 52–59.

WIENER, L., THEUT, S., STEINBERG, S., RIEKERT, K. and PIZZO, P. (1994) 'The HIV infected child: parental responses and psychosocial implications', *American Journal of Orthopsychiatry*, **64**, 3, pp. 485–92.

WOLTERS, P., BROUWERS, P., MOSS, H. and PIZZO, P. (1995) 'Differential receptive and expressive language functioning of children and symptomatic HIV disease and relation to CT scan brain abnormlities', *Pediatrics*, **95**, 1, pp. 112–19.

Chapter 4

The Impact of HIV Infection on Partners and Relatives

Barbara Hedge

HIV infection has impact not only on those living with HIV, but also on infected partners and relatives. In this chapter the consequences for affected partners of people with HIV infection are discussed, in terms of their roles, duties and concerns, their needs and coping strategies and the emotional consequences. The effects on other relatives, in particular parents, is also reviewed, together with the range of forms of support for partners and families, including the role of health and social services as well as that of voluntary and non-governmental organizations.

Introduction

HIV disease does not only impact on the infected person; there is evidence that partners, family members and other close individuals are also affected, often negatively. Interestingly, most of the studies on partners and families of people with HIV disease report the effects on the 'caregivers', automatically assigning to partners and families a role usually associated with the care of the very young, the infirm or the elderly. However, many people infected with HIV are well for many years, so the psychological impact may begin before and last longer than any physical caregiving. Powell-Cope (1995) found that in couples where one person had HIV, both partners perceived infection as causing a major life transition as both were confronted by multiple losses, including the possible death of the person with HIV and hence the relationship, the loss of health, independence, intimacy and privacy. Partners or relatives may also have to cope with stress relating to the stigma attached to homophobia or illegal drug use.

HIV disease presents extreme challenges to primary caregivers, especially partners infected with HIV; they may need to adjust to the care recipient's disease progression, manage role conflict in the relationship and fatigue (Folkman, Chesney and Christopher-Richards, 1994). Partners, friends and families are in a position to provide persons with HIV with a wide range of valued resources, including emotional support, companionship, information and advice, task assistance, and material aid which may significantly enhance quality of life. Unfortunately, many factors frequently interfere with the degree to which friends and family members *actually* provide effective support.

This chapter attempts to explore the impact of HIV disease on partners and families of people with HIV disease and suggests ways in which they might cope effectively with practical and emotional issues.

Partners

In the Western world the vast majority of people with HIV are young gay men. For most of these men, the primary caregiver is their partner, also a young gay man (Turner and Catania, 1997). In this respect, HIV disease is atypical; for most illnesses the burden of care is met by families, with the typical carer being a middle-aged, female relative. This means that there are few role models for partners of gay men with HIV disease and little societal support. Frequently gay relationships are not recognized legally. This can result in difficulties about housing, should a gay man die without a will or inadequately insured. The difficulties faced by gay men with sick partners may not be formally recognized at work and they may not be afforded the privileges such as time off, usually granted to the spouses of people who are terminally ill.

McCann and Wadsworth (1992) found that only 8 per cent of gay men with AIDS identified a parent or sibling to be their primary carer. For some it may be that the family is negative and rejecting, leaving the partner and friends to be the principal supporters. For others the family may not know of the HIV infection, so it is unable to offer support. This is not uncommon as many people with HIV disease try to protect their families from the stigma, hostility, prejudice and rejection they associate with HIV. Families may not be aware of their child's sexuality, sexual behaviours or drug use. It is also more usual for adults to be living with their partner of choice, and if necessary, cared for by them; what is novel is for there to be so many same-sex young couples in which at least one person has a potentially fatal illness that may require high levels of physical and emotional support.

Roles, Duties and Concerns

Being the partner of a person with HIV disease is neither a simple nor a singular task. The diseases which mark advanced HIV disease are increasingly cared for at home. Thus the partner being the closest person usually becomes the primary caregiver. Hays, Magee and Chauncey (1994) discuss helpful behaviours identified by a group of gay men with AIDS. Most important were the provision of love and concern, being a confidant, providing encouragement and offering proactive assistance. When offering support, the implicit meaning of the offer needs to be considered; for example, does it convey a message that the person cannot be responsible for their self-care or for decision making, or a message that despite infection the person with AIDS still has opportunities to reciprocate support? Support can easily be declined or psychological distress increased if such messages are received at the wrong time or given in the wrong way. To be effective the partner needs to have the sensitivity of a trained counsellor as well as having sufficient time and energy in which to provide support. The responsibilities of partners often include helping with the everyday practicalities of having HIV disease, such as ensuring that the recommended medication is taken or assisting with complicated medication regimens. However, even when people with HIV disease are asymptomatic and well, the awareness that their illness is likely to be fatal but has no definite time span can lower mood. Partners are often involved in helping to maintain motivation and encourage the use of active coping strategies in people with HIV disease.

As well as giving support, partners have to cope with the reality of their own losses as they see physical and maybe mental deterioration in the people they love, changes in their relationships and uncertain futures. They may have to cope with anticipated grief as they recognize that partners are dying. These tasks have to be accomplished without the support they would normally use – the support of their partner. Frequently an HIV negative partner becomes the principal caregiver and family manager, particularly when the person with HIV becomes symptomatic. He or she may become the main economic provider. If these roles do not mirror those in the relationship before HIV disease, this change can lead to upset and disturbance in a couple.

The uncertainty attached to the course of disease can also cause practical difficulties for carers. It is not easy to predict when a person might require full-time care. Even if an employer is willing to support a partner by offering long-term leave, this is difficult to do when it cannot be planned in advance. For many couples, the partners who have become the main financial support have to face the difficult decision of whether to continue working and leave the care of the sick person to others, or to abandon financial independence and maybe their career in order to care for their partners. With increasing advances in efficacious medication (Palella *et al.*, 1998) it is possible that a person with HIV disease may swing a number of times from needing a large amount of care to being well and independent. Although many employers and many individual carers can cope with one period of time spent away from work, it is less likely that most can withstand several unplanned spells of absence.

Intuitively, it might be thought that severity of illness would be related to increased caregiving burden. However, a review of studies examining care for the elderly (Woods and Britton, 1985) found no link between the two. Some studies showed that it was specific problem behaviours such as frequent demands for attention which were related to increased burden of care. Although Pakenham, Dadds and Terry (1994, 1995) found that carers of people with symptomatic HIV disease were more distressed than carers of asymptomatic people, they found no association between symptomatology and caregiving burden. It may be that more detailed studies are required to see how partners are affected by problem behaviours, e.g. those brought about by HIV-related brain impairment or the psychiatric manifestations of disease.

Medication Issues

The recent widespread introduction of highly active antiretroviral therapies has improved the length of life and the quality of life for many people with HIV disease (Palella *et al.*, 1998). Improvement in a person's health can be an unexpectedly difficult time for partners. Most relationships involve some role diversification, even if not along traditional lines. In times of need, such as during severe illness, people can alter their roles quite quickly. However, it can be more difficult to revert to previous patterns of living when health improves. Such changes can have an immense effect on a partner who may psychologically have been preparing for a person's death. It can be difficult to readjust to expecting an individual to have a reasonable quality of life, to be contemplating a return to work, to enjoy sex once more and to be ready to take up some of the roles and duties of home life. This can be particularly difficult in illnesses such as HIV disease where the long-term prognosis remains uncertain. For example, Brown and Smith (1992) reported how many wives of men who had experienced a myocardial infarction became overprotective of their husbands.

An additional stress can be the knowledge that currently only a limited number of antiretroviral drug combinations are available. As intolerance or drug resistance is encountered, people advance to different drug combinations. They fear approaching the day when their virus is resistant to all known antiretrovirals drugs. The psychological effect of these medically beneficial new therapies on partners remains to be documented.

Dealing with the Relationship

Seeing physical or emotional changes due to HIV disease in a person one cares about can be deeply distressing. Not surprisingly, HIV has an effect on most couples' relationships. Some couples try to maintain their relationships by avoiding the issue of HIV. Although this may help in the short term, it can lead to individuals feeling very unsupported. Partners may avoid expressing their concerns about HIV or enquiring about the emotional impact of a patient's illness. If these issues are not addressed, the person with HIV may surmise that the fact he has HIV has no effect on his partner, and interpret this as indicating a lack of love or concern. If the person with HIV dies with important issues remaining unresolved or important messages remaining unsaid, complicated bereavements may follow. Consequently, partners have to be aware of the fine balance which needs to be drawn between the amount of concern they express and the amount they indicate they can cope with.

Communication

Discussing difficult but important issues is always hard (Perakyla and Bor, 1990). Paradoxically, it is often more of a problem in couples who are very fond of each other; neither partner wants to distress the other, so difficult issues are avoided, e.g. safer sex, planning for the future, dying, power of attorney, wills and funerals. Postponement does not ease the situation; it can increase stress levels as each tries to guess the other's views from outward signs such as their demeanour and behaviour.

Although honest, open communication is generally beneficial to a relationship, it is possible to spend too much time discussing HIV-related issues. If HIV becomes the sole focus of a relationship, it can limit the time available for activities which make life enjoyable and which support the relationship. Couples can find it difficult to decide how much time to devote to each other. Because they fear there may be little time left, they may try to spend every minute together. However, if this is not the life pattern that they enjoyed pre-HIV, it is unlikely to meet their needs and may produce conflict.

Sexual Functioning

Sexual difficulties have been widely reported in people with HIV disease and their partners (Catalán et al., 1992; Klimes et al., 1992; George, 1990). People infected with HIV are usually very keen to protect their sexual partners from acquiring HIV, and partners who are HIV negative are usually keen to remain so.

Discussing safer sex can be disturbing, even with a regular partner who knows of the infection, as it is a reminder of the risks of infection, illness and death. Such thoughts may reduce sexual desire and induce fears of sexual expression. This can lead to the avoidance of any physical contact in case it leads to a sexual encounter. Signs of love and affection such as touching, hugging and kissing are all boosts to a person's self-esteem. The withdrawal of these signs may leave a person feeling they are worthless, and may result in lowered mood and diminished quality of life.

Sexual dysfunction has been widely reported in people with AIDS. It can be a consequence of hormone imbalance, depressed libido associated with severe disease, depression or fear of transmitting or catching HIV. So it is not unusual to encounter difficulties in either people with HIV or their partners. If partners do not address the problem, it is very easy for the withdrawal of physical affection to be misinterpreted. The person denied physical comfort may feel unattractive and not valued. This can be very undermining in any relationship. Often a simple statement of sexual desires and concerns is sufficient for a couple to start discussing their feelings and safer sexual options, and to renew their sex life.

Organic Brain Disorder

HIV related brain disorder is not uncommon in the later stages of HIV disease with AIDS dementia occurring in 12–15 per cent of people with HIV infection and cognitive impairment being demonstrable in up to 30 per cent of individuals. The prevalence of central nervous system involvement does seem to be decreasing with the advent of combination antiretroviral medications, although this clinical impression still has to be demonstrated by controlled trials.

High dose zidovudine is associated with improvements in neuropsychological well-being and there are indications that improvements in cognitive functioning may be associated with some of the newer antiretroviral drugs. There still remain individuals in whom cognitive and behavioural changes may be seen which cannot be reversed. In some cases the cognitive dysfunction is a result of major depression; mood dysfunction and organic disease sometimes coexist. Although the differentiation of organic disease from functional disease may be difficult, the problems presented to the carer may be similar. Care of those who are severely disturbed can be onerous. Provision of social and community support for the carers, family and friends is of great importance (Ostrow, Grant and Atkinson, 1988). If residential care is not available or is not desired by the partner, family or caregivers then attendance at day centres and intermittent respite care can help to maintain an individual in the community.

Emotional Impact

Caregiving is significantly associated with psychological distress in many illnesses (Rabins *et al.*, 1990). Even so, Raveis and Siegel (1991) argue that caring for a partner with HIV is unique and is more intensely stressful than caring for a person with other diseases. Irving, Bor and Catalán (1995) showed 45 per cent of partners of men with AIDS were 'definite psychiatric cases' whereas 21 per cent were 'probable psychiatric cases'. Coyle (1993) found a rate of 29 per cent of psychiatric cases in a UK community sample of gay men and Grey and Hedge (1998) found 54 per cent of psychiatric cases in a sample of partners of gay men with HIV disease at varying stages of disease progression. So despite advances in treatment and more therapeutic optimism in recent years, high levels of distress are still seen in people's partners.

As HIV disease progresses, the caring responsibilities of a partner can increase. People can become physically and mentally exhausted, especially if they have not sought out or been in a position to receive support from others, e.g. friends or families. A number of studies have described the challenges faced by these caregivers (McCann and Wadsworth, 1992; M.A. Brown and Powell-Cope, 1993; Folkman *et al.*, 1994; Wrubel and Folkman, 1997). Most research has focused solely on carers of people with AIDS, although distress has been found in partners of people at all stages of HIV infection (Grey and

Hedge, 1999). Laurichesse *et al.* (1998) found that 5 per cent of patients died before progressing to AIDS. This could mean that significant rates of distress or unmet needs in partners of people with asymptomatic HIV disease are being missed.

Studies do not agree as to whether illness severity increases distress in partners. Pakenham, Dadds and Terry (1995) found illness severity not to increase the burden and distress for partners of people with AIDS, whereas Grey and Hedge (1998) did find an association between the partner's perception of the patient's health and the distress experienced; the worse the health, the greater the distress.

It is well documented in the study of older adults that lower levels of marital or familial intimacy are associated with higher perceived levels of caregiver burden (Morris, Morris and Britton, 1988; Gilleard *et al.*, 1984), as evidenced in higher levels of reported strain and depression. Similarly, in studies of partners of gay men with AIDS, Folkman and co-workers (Folkman, Chesney and Christopher-Richards, 1984; Folkman *et al.*, 1984) found that the caregiver burden was influenced by the quality of the relationship and related to distress. Satisfaction with social support was linked with low levels of distress (Grey and Hedge, 1998).

Anger is a common response to having HIV. People with HIV may turn the anger on themselves and exhibit self-destructive behaviours, e.g. not taking their medications as prescribed, not taking care of themselves, not sleeping adequately, or indulging in excessive alcohol or drug use. Seeing such maladaptive behaviours can be distressing even when partners can recognize and understand the cause, i.e. the uncontrollability of living with HIV. It can be more distressing for partners when the emotions are turned outward. Partners can find that whatever they do to help and support is not sufficient; they are constantly criticized in a very personal way. The difficulty is that nothing the partner, or anyone, can do is what the person with HIV wants, i.e. to turn back the clock, to take away the virus. Emotions of anger, guilt, hatred, sadness and frustration may all be dissipated. Ironically, partners frequently bear the brunt of emotional outbursts. It seems that people find it easiest to vent emotions on those they trust to support and stay with them. Thus, partners and close family members often experience the most difficult aspects of the behaviours of people with HIV.

Even when partners understand that people with HIV can misdirect their feelings, it can be difficult to cope with the emotions raised, such as feelings of inadequacy, the fear of a lack of reciprocated love, or anger that the support given freely is not recognized or appreciated. In some cases partners have responded by saying they wished the person would just die. They then become guilt-ridden, having only meant that they wanted the awful situation to cease. Both partners may become distressed with neither having anyone to give comfort.

Folkman (1997) in a longitudinal study of the experiences of partners while caring for men with AIDS through illness and death, reported high levels of depression, particularly around the time of a partner's death. Interestingly, this study found that the partners also experienced high positive affects, which Folkman suggests are the outcome of successful coping. For example, the distress associated with a dying partner can be coped with by positive reinterpretation. By assigning positive meanings to events which happen, such as a smile or enjoying a day in a sunny garden, partners can generate positive mood states which aid in coping with the terrible reality.

Caring for a partner, especially when young, can be particularly grievous. Many stressors that are associated with increased suicide risk in the general population, e.g. life events, depression, social isolation and cumulative stress, are seen in the partners of people with HIV (G.W. Brown, 1979; Paykel, Prusoff and Myers, 1975; Schneider *et al.*, 1991; Slater and Depue, 1981). Rosengard and Folkman (1997) report 53 per cent of gay or bisexual male caregivers of partners with AIDS to report suicide ideation. Thoughts of suicide just prior to and immediately following the death of the partner are related to the perception of greater caregiver burden, poor social support and the use of ineffectual coping strategies such as behavioural escape avoidance.

Bereavement

It is well documented that the psychological effects of caregiving and bereavement can be intense and long-lasting and are often associated with increased distress in partners and close relatives (Middleton *et al.*, 1997). Lennon, Martin and Dean (1990) found the intensity of grief during bereavement to be related to the involvement in caretaking during end-stage disease and to the adequacy of practical and emotional support given to the caregiver during this time. Suicide ideation is associated with bereavement in the general population (Stroebe and Stroebe, 1993). Most studies of suicide ideation in the bereaved consider samples of those most commonly bereaved, i.e. those over 65 years of age. The few studies that look at the effects on younger age groups suggest that young males may be especially vulnerable (Stroebe and Stroebe, 1983).

Suicide ideation is common in caregivers of people with HIV disease; Rosengard and Folkman (1997) found 55 per cent of caregivers to report suicide ideation at some time during their two-year study. For the bereaved, suicide ideation was associated with increased caregiver burden, less perceived social support, less social integration and greater reliance on behavioural escape-avoidance coping strategies. Those who were optimistic in outlook seemed to have some measure of protection.

Suicidal ideation has been shown to be more prevalent in bereaved caregivers than in those who are not bereaved (Lennon, Martin and Dean, 1990). Richmond and Ross (1994) examined patterns of bereavement in partners and family members of people who had died of AIDS-related illnesses. Most described feelings of loneliness and emptiness. Self-euthanasia generated ambivalent feelings. Many received support from friends, support groups or professional counsellors rather than from family members. The death of a person with AIDS is often a time when care services that could provide some support to partners are withdrawn. It is important that HIV services acknowledge the needs of partners at this time and provide support when necessary.

Multiple Losses

The phenomenon of multiple loss due to HIV disease has been reported in many studies. Dean, Hall and Martin (1988) studied patterns of bereavement in gay men in New York; they found that 95 per cent of the sample had experienced HIV-related losses with an average of 6.2 HIV-related deaths each. McKusick (1991) reported a similar cohort in San Francisco to experience increased distress involving psychological and emotional numbness, shrinking away from friends and resources, increased symptoms of complicated bereavement (inordinate guilt, calcified anger, rage, indifference) and more depression as more people with HIV died. More recently, Martin (1998) reported a direct dose–response relationship between the number of bereavement episodes experienced and the onset of traumatic stress response symptoms. No association was seen between bereavement and problem drinking or drug use, but bereavement was associated with more sedative and recreational drug use. These studies obviously include many people whose partners are infected with HIV, hence they suggest that previous experience with HIV-related loss might be an important moderating variable of distress in individuals affected by HIV disease in a partner.

A background of multiple HIV-related losses could well influence the coping skills, motivation and ability of a partner to access the resources necessary to decrease caregiver burden or to suggest adaptive coping skills. Schwartzberg (1992) suggested that the experience of many friends dying may make grief more complicated, and with their partner's death some generate feelings of survivor guilt.

The HIV Positive Partner

Providing care to an individual who has a potentially terminal illness is stressful; more so if the carer has the same disease when they have a constant example of how living and dying might be for them. The difference is that they will probably have to cope alone. Lynn and Silverman (1996) in a US sample reported 36 per cent of caregivers to people with symptomatic HIV disease to be themselves HIV positive. Although there were no differences in health between the HIV positive and HIV negative caregivers, those who were positive perceived their health to be worse and reported more health-related distress. Folkman *et al.* (1996) found that carers who were positive and in long relationships reported more daily hassles in their lives and tended to use distancing and self-blame in order to cope. These did not appear to be successful coping strategies as they were associated with unrelieved depressive mood. Rosengard and Folkman (1997) found that HIV positive caregivers were not more likely than HIV negative caregivers to report suicide ideation.

Folkman *et al.* (1992) described the experiences of caregivers to people with HIV during their illnesses and after their deaths. Prior to the death of partners, HIV positive caregivers were less distressed than those not infected, whereas after death the infected partners showed more distress. A possible explanation is that those who were infected viewed the experience as a model for their own death. First they empathized with the patient; after the death they experienced increased awareness of their own mortality. Martin and Dean (1993) suggested that partners realize they will face a similar experience alone as their own infection makes it less likely they will find a new partner. There is also some evidence that physical health can be affected by the death of a partner. Kemeny *et al.* (1995) reported the immune system to change in ways that are relevant to HIV progression after the death of an intimate partner.

Most of the studies where both partners are infected with HIV dichotomize the couple into sick person and carer. In many couples this is justifiable. Increasingly though, as antiretroviral treatments start earlier and people live longer, we are seeing many couples in which both partners are generally well, are having regular medical check-ups and are on combinations of antiretroviral medications. The roles of the sick person and the carer have become blurred and may switch according to need. Although HIV disease now has many characteristics of a chronic disease, uncertainty about the efficacy of current antiretroviral regimens in the face of drug resistance has maintained the anxiety typically associated with acute potentially fatal illnesses – the fear that treatment will become ineffectual and that ill health will follow. We have still to investigate the issues for couples who do not fit the traditional model of sick person and carer.

Coping

How do people cope with caring for a person with HIV disease? The coping strategies are interesting as, to some extent, they are amenable to change (Chesney, Folkman and Chambers, 1996). Few studies have investigated the coping strategies used. In an Australian study of the caregiving partners, family and friends of people with HIV disease, Pakenham, Dadds and Terry (1995) found the absence of psychological distress to be associated with the use of problem-focused coping. In a US sample of gay men whose partners had AIDS, Folkman *et al.* (1994) found the caregiving burden to be at its minimum when the partners used coping strategies of active problem solving, distancing, cognitive escape avoidance and seeking social support. Grey and Hedge (1998) found the most anxious partners of people at all stages of HIV disease to use a large number of coping strategies. One possible explanation for this is that by using a large number of coping strategies, none can be used effectively and anxiety remains. An alternative explanation is that those who were most anxious were using as many coping strategies as they could in an attempt to ameliorate the situation. The highest distress was seen in people using behavioural and mental disengagement. Avoidance of problems by disengagement may provide short-term relief but does not help in the long term.

Suppression of competing activities is also related to higher levels of distress (Wacholder, 1993; Grey and Hedge, 1998). This has been described as an effective way of coping (Carver *et al.*, 1989). However, when caring for a person with HIV disease, it could be that the patient becomes exclusively the centre and focus of life, at the expense of the partner's own needs. This strategy may prove beneficial at certain times of stress, e.g. during an acute hospital admission, but it is rarely sustainable over longer periods of time. This is supported by Rosengard and Folkman (1997), who found that greater use of behavioural escape-avoidance coping strategies was associated with recent suicide ideation. Moskowitz *et al.* (1996) found that people used more problem-focused types of coping and more cognitive escape avoidance during caregiving than during bereavement; this suggests the tasks to be dealt with before and after a partner's death are very different. Before the death, partners seem able to address the issues of living by using problem-focused coping strategies, but they find it difficult to address the associated cognitions, i.e. deal mentally with the reality of the situation. Positive reappraisal appeared to mediate distress.

One of the problems with most of these studies is that many are cross-sectional, i.e. many are snapshots of how a partner is coping at a particular time. Longitudinal studies are required to investigate the rise or fall of distress levels when a particular strategy is used over a long period of time.

Needs of Partners

Partners of people with HIV disease have needs that extend beyond practical support at times of illness. This is not to discount the importance of practical issues, e.g. providing companionship and task assistance to ease the burden of caregiving; it is to acknowledge that the psychological distress associated with loving a person with a potentially fatal illness can be immense, even when that person is well. As long as there remains uncertainty in the prognosis for people with HIV disease and in the efficacy and longevity of available medications, distress levels are bound to remain high.

The difficulties they face indicate that, besides the individuals infected with HIV, partners too may benefit from individual psychological support which aims to enhance adaptive coping strategies, communication and assertiveness skills, and to tackle psychological distress. The intensity of distress reported shows the need for a forum in which the topic of suicide can be raised, and opportunities allowed for the discussion of associated thoughts and feelings. Adaptive coping strategies may be needed to reframe suicidal thoughts. Difficulties which directly affect the couple, e.g. communication or sexual problems, may require psychological support for both the person with HIV disease and the partner.

Finally, the needs of bereaved partners should not be forgotten. Although grief reactions are a normal response to death, the possible isolation of people whose partners have died from an AIDS-related illness and the effects of multiple bereavements in societies affected by HIV disease, increase the chances of pathological grief reactions. The need for partners to have easy access to bereavement counselling is most important.

Families

This section considers the families of adults with HIV disease. The specific needs of people with HIV disease that relate to the desires for a child or issues related to having young children are considered in Chapter 3.

A family member can only be supportive to a person with HIV disease if aware of the issues. In a US study investigating awareness of HIV by parents and siblings in heterosexual discordant couples, Foley *et al.* (1994) reported 78 per cent of HIV positive women and 40 per cent of HIV positive men to have told their mother of their HIV status. Awareness did not necessarily lead to support; 25 per cent of HIV positive partners and nearly 50 per cent of HIV negative partners had no support. Lack of support was particularly marked for African-American partners. In a San Francisco cohort of gay and bisexual men, Stemple (1995) found that within one year of a positive HIV test only 37 per cent had told a family member. Even fewer, only 35 per cent of their male negative partners and 28 per cent of their female negative partners, had told their mothers.

Family awareness increased as disease progressed, many couples delaying disclosure until the person with HIV disease became hospitalized, had an altered physical appearance, became severely depressed or exhibited behaviours which suggested HIV brain disease. Disclosure is often delayed as people not only fear judgement of their lifestyles which resulted in the acquisition of HIV but also dread possible stigma as others fear contagion and fear the negative emotions – anxiety, grief and anger – of those they tell. Compared with positive partners, negative partners were less likely to have members of their own family providing support.

Disclosure to a family member was negatively associated with the level of education obtained, i.e. those with most education were least likely to have informed a close family member. This could reflect less need, a greater sense of control, a greater desire or ability to manage on their own or with friends, a greater fear of embarrassment or other emotion, or less willingness to test rejection.

Difficulties Faced by Parents

There is little documented in the HIV literature about the difficulties parents face when knowing that their (adult) child has HIV disease. Many parents talk of the unnatural order of events encountered when a parent has to face burying their own child. Frequently parents question whether they are to blame for the HIV infection, suggesting that the upbringing they gave their children may have resulted in them becoming drug users, gay or indiscriminate in their choice of sexual partners. Even when they profess to understanding little about the lifestyles of their offspring, they rarely abandon them. McGinn (1996) examined the impact of an HIV positive adult living with parents in a rural area in the American Midwest. HIV stigma caused more difficulties to the parents than the physical and mental care they had to provide. Parents had few places or people to whom they could turn when dealing with the consequences of an adult child with HIV status. The importance of establishing contact with others in similar situations is particularly important when HIV remains a close family secret. Although this can be a wise option when stigma and discrimination are feared, the psychological impact of containing the secret without support can be immense. It may be associated with complicated bereavement if their child should die.

Support for Partners and Families

Distress in the partners of people with HIV is common and may be severe. The emotional needs of partners can be supported by professional individuals, e.g. clinical psychologists or trained counsellors. Many services for people with HIV disease recognize this need and provide for the mental health support of partners. When the needs of partners are met, they are often more able to cope with the difficulties of the person with HIV themselves and thus reduce the burden on the health service.

Information Networks

Over the last few years information about HIV disease has become widely available in hospital leaflets, the gay press and publications aimed specifically at people with HIV. Many of these and other sources of information are available via the Internet. Directing partners towards publications which address their particular needs will not only keep them abreast of the latest findings in the management of HIV disease but also empower them by enabling them to take responsibility for accessing pertinent information.

Recognition of the Dual Needs of Partners and Families

Partners and families of people with HIV have a dual task. Firstly, they usually want to support the person they love, practically and emotionally. Secondly they have to cope with their emotional reactions which are responses to being close to a person with a potentially fatal illness. For partners or relatives who are themselves HIV positive there are also the thoughts and feelings raised by their own infection. Managing these tasks simultaneously or deciding on priorities can increase distress. Support from an outsider, who can be both objective and empathic, whether a professional carer or a voluntary worker, can often help people to make realistic decisions. For example, when a person is unwell the partner may not know whether to resign from paid employment in order to provide care, whether to engage a nurse or to send the person with HIV to an inpatient care centre. The indecision can often cause more distress than acting on any of the possible options.

Access to services, e.g. clinical psychology, can often prevent psychological distress by helping partners and families to develop appropriate coping skills before they need to be used. Partners and families can be relieved when they are allowed to talk about the realities of the situation away from the sick person and realize that they are not expected to cope alone. Support with problem solving, prioritization and time management can enable them to devote time for themselves and can empower them to continue with the minimum of stress. It is not empowering for health care workers to cope *for* them. Too much or inappropriate support can increase psychological distress and lower self-esteem as the person interprets the support as indicating that they are unable to cope and meet the needs of their loved one.

Coping with the Negative Emotions of a Person with HIV Disease

Therapeutic support may usefully deal directly with symptoms such as anxiety, depression, guilt, fear and low self-esteem through cognitive-behavioural interventions. Such symptoms can be exacerbated in partners and families by the emotional reactions of the individuals with HIV infection. Advice concerning the appropriateness of referrals to mental health professionals, such as psychiatrists or clinical psychologists, and some training in empathic assertiveness may empower the partner to guide the person with HIV towards an appropriate professional. Such referrals are then beneficial to both.

Partners can be reassured by the knowledge that emotional outbursts directed towards those they love are not uncommon in people with HIV. In order to cope with these negative emotions, partners can be schooled in appropriate responses which help the person with HIV to express emotions and cope with the issues raised in more productive ways (Table 4.1). Involving the partner or close family member in the psychological support of a person

Table 4.1 *Coping with negative emotions in the person with HIV disease*

1. Allow, even encourage, venting of emotions.
2. Acknowledge the feelings of the person with HIV:
    It isn't fair.
    It is difficult.
3. Direct into a positive, coping framework:
    So, what shall we do about it?
4. After the event, discuss the benefit of talking about feelings.
5. Discuss the difficulties of receiving emotional outbursts.
6. Indicate how you will react the next time such a behaviour occurs:
    Okay, I know that's difficult.
    How do you feel?
    Go on, what else is troubling you?
    Let's hear everything, then we can see what needs attention first.
7. Suggest alternative modes of expressions.

with HIV is not only a cost-effective way in which to help the person with HIV, but also enables the partner to distance himself from negative personal remarks and retain a sense of self-worth.

In some areas there exist networks of 'buddies'. Buddies are people who are willing and able to support a person with HIV disease (often those with an AIDS diagnosis) in a number of ways. If the person with HIV is no longer working, or spends many hours alone or with only the partner, a buddy can be a useful addition to a support network. Partners can encourage the use of a buddy to prevent isolation and to contribute to the provision of emotional or practical support for the person with HIV.

Emotional Support

Therapeutic support may usefully deal directly with symptoms such as anger, anxiety, depression, guilt, fear and low self-esteem through cognitive-behavioural interventions. Ways of coping with expected and unexpected losses, fears of being inadequate, and inappropriate coping strategies such as excessive alcohol or drug use can usefully be addressed in similar ways to those described in Chapter 8.

Practical Support

There is a clear need for practical support. This can range from needing some occasional help while a sick person is being cared for, e.g. help with household chores, to requiring full-time support for care at the end of a person's life. Partners and families caring for a person with HIV disease often think in black and white terms and only look for all or nothing solutions. In fact, it is better to consider a wide range of practical support options. Here the acute centre counsellor or social worker may be able to provide direct advice or put partners in contact with organizers of services who can then take over detailed support planning. For those living in areas with a high incidence of HIV infection, practical support is usually available. Unfortunately, some services for people with HIV have been reduced or closed in order to pay for expensive antiretroviral medications. As these are not 100 per cent efficacious, this has increased the burden on remaining care centres.

Partners need to be advised about community care teams, the availability of day care and respite care facilities. The use of specialized day care can enable a person to continue working and remain financially solvent while being confident that their partner is well cared for. Being able to have a personal life as well as caring for a sick person does increase the sense of well-being and quality of life in partners (Grey and Hedge, 1998). It may well have a secondary effect on the person with HIV who does not need to feel guilty about being the cause of psychological distress or low mood in their partner.

Caring for a sick person all the time can be very demanding. Some partners or families prefer to take on this task themselves rather than use other care facilities. In order to be able to continue providing high quality care, even the most dedicated carers require rests. It is often possible to make arrangements with residential care centres for a person to receive intermittent respite care for short periods of time on a regular basis, e.g. one week in every six. This allows the carers to have a break and remain caring for a much longer period of time.

When high levels of care are needed, it is often useful to involve professional or volunteer care workers in the arrangements. Not only are they knowledgeable about local services, but they understand the huge effort, emotional and physical, which may be involved in the provision of care. Untrained family and friends are often well meaning but have no conception of the effort needed to provide high quality care to someone who requires help with taking medications, washing, toileting and feeding. They may then lose the ability to be a good friend, lover or relative – roles that can never be played by the health carers.

The need for practical support can be particularly necessary when the person with HIV disease has a concurrent psychiatric disorder or organic brain disorder. It can be useful to have a power of attorney arranged before it is likely to be needed. Access to legal services needs to be set up while the person retains good cognitive faculties and has no severe mental health disorder. Before a couple or a family can set up such a system, they must be able to communicate realistically about their views on various treatment, financial and end-of-life situations. Discussing these issues can be distressing in the short term. In the long term, distress is usually reduced when both the person with HIV and the partner or chosen family member can relax, knowing that if cognitive or mental health problems occur, the wishes of the person with HIV will be respected.

This highlights the importance of establishing effective communication early in the disease. The need for practical support in these circumstances is likely to be obvious. It needs to be remembered that partners and families may experience the cognitive and mental and physical changes in the person with HIV as the loss of the person they have known and loved. They may be anticipating the person's death. The provision of emotional support at this time should not be overlooked.

Sex

The inability to continue with a satisfactory sex life can be upsetting both to people with HIV and their partners. Although there may be irreversible organic damage, it is important that couples do not assume this and forego appropriate examinations and investigations. In many cases sexual dysfunction is the result of depression, anxiety or low self-esteem. Treatment of a concurrent mood disorder may improve sexual functioning. When dysfunction is the result of anxieties concerning the possible transmission of HIV in either the person with HIV or the partner, it can be helpful to improve communication skills between the couple together with cognitive behaviour therapy to address realistic and irrational cognitions.

End-of-Life Issues and Bereavement

Despite the revolutionary new antiretroviral treatments now available, people with HIV disease do still die of AIDS-related illnesses. Giving prognoses of times of death except in very general terms is not helpful. Neither is giving undue reassurance that all will be well. Although it is difficult to live with uncertainty, being able to do this is beneficial. Partners and families can benefit from knowing that the time of death is probably close. If there are queries as to whether it is time to say goodbye, it is useful to encourage people to say everything they wish to now. There is no harm in saying goodbye again at a later date if the person lives longer than expected. Coping with a death is never easy. However caring a person may have been, retrospectively they always feel they could have done or said more.

It is important to allow recently bereaved people to talk about a death, express distress and take time to cope with its reality (Chapter 8). Health care workers can themselves become distressed in a response to a bereaved person's distress and summon a mental health professional prematurely. If, as time goes by, the normal tasks of bereavement are not managed and there is no change from the acute distress experienced at the time of death, then bereavement counselling can be useful.

AIDS-related bereavement can involve many losses. If partners have not been accepted by the family of the person with HIV, they may be excluded from funerals or the final arrangements. In order to secure the rights of partners at this time, it is useful to have drawn up specifications for the arrangements at an earlier date and incorporated them into a will. The need for a will is particularly important for unmarried couples (e.g. gay men). If a person dies intestate, their next of kin is likely to be a biological relative. When funeral arrangements and inheritance of possessions has not been specified in a will, surviving partners may find they are left with little. It is not unknown for partners to lose their home and all joint possessions (Doka, 1987).

Systems of Support

The first line of support for partners and families is often other relatives or friends. When this support is absent or insufficient to meet the needs of partners and families, external support can be provided by the acute centre where the person with HIV is receiving specialist care, in a primary care setting or by voluntary organizations.

When the partner or family is being seen in the same setting as the person with HIV disease, care must be taken to respect the privacy of all concerned. Everyone has the right to confidentiality whether they are the patient, the partner or the parents. Breaking confidentiality, even to well-meaning parents, usually does not solve any problems. The person whose confidentiality has been broken may find it difficult to trust the care person further and may be less likely to disclose important or emotionally difficult information in the future. When confidentiality is respected, there is less reason for difficulties to be hidden and for problems to remain unresolved (Pinching, 1994).

After a person with HIV has died, some partners or families find it difficult to revisit the place where their loved one died or was very sick. This highlights the need for flexibility of access to bereavement services. The task of the psychologist or the social worker in the acute hospital or hospice is often to put partners and families in touch with other, maybe local services for bereavement work rather than to continue the care themselves. This is not always possible. When severely disturbed, the bereaved may require more specialized care than is available in the community. People who live in a region with a low incidence of HIV may find few services for people with HIV, and even fewer for bereaved partners or families.

Individual Therapy

Many partners are offered individual psychological support by a clinical psychologist or trained counsellor. This can usefully address the emotional needs of the partner. It can also increase the use of problem solving, bring about changes in the coping strategies used and consider specific issues such as maintaining safer sex, and telling friends and relatives about HIV. Many issues are similar to those confronted by people with HIV, and similar therapeutic approaches can be used (Catalán, Burgess and Klimes, 1995); see Chapter 8.

Couple Therapy

When both the person with HIV and the partner have difficulties, couple therapy can be considered (Ussher, 1990). This is particularly useful when there are communication difficulties within the couple. Role-playing alternative ways of communicating and joint exploration of the feelings attached to communications can be beneficial. The couple may also address sexual dysfunction together. Even if only one person in a couple requests help with sexual difficulties, it can be useful to see both partners as sex is usually interactive. Both partners may need to change their behaviours in order to achieve a successful experience. As sexual difficulties are often an outward sign of complex relationship problems, it is useful to provide some time when each person can talk privately and confidentially about the relationship with the therapist.

Groups

Folkman, Chesney and Christopher-Richards (1994) found that caregivers sustained positive morale by deriving meaning from their caregiving. One way to capitalize on this is by involving carers in self-help groups. Through groups, carers can derive benefit by sharing information and coping experiences with others, thus increasing their morale, and by being the recipient of similar support from others. Health professionals are in a good position to organize and facilitate groups.

Groups with many different remits have proved beneficial to partners of people with HIV disease. Gazarik and Fischman (1995) reported on a 12-week group for the infected person and their partner. The group primarily focused on couples' issues, individual concerns, conflicts, and experiences relating to the HIV diagnosis such as loss, redefinition of roles and denial; it was judged beneficial. Hedge and Glover (1990) were keen to provide a forum in which both people with HIV and partners of people with HIV could speak freely of difficulties they were encountering without fear of upsetting their partners. Couples were recruited to join a mixed group so that both points of view could be presented. However, only one person from each couple could attend. The group enabled people with HIV to make suggestions for models of care to partners in a non-personal setting, and its usefulness was highly rated by all attenders.

Most people with HIV disease live in metropolitan areas that are relatively well provided with dedicated facilities. However, their parents and relatives may be scattered all over the county in both rural and urban locations. Those in or near large towns may be able to access individual support at local HIV care centres or find parent support groups in the community. Those in rural areas will almost certainly find nothing locally. A voluntary organization, such as the Terence Higgins Trust in the United Kingdom, may be able to put parents in contact with others in their own area. In some places, parents have developed highly active groups that support their own needs and those of their children.

Summary

The impact of HIV infection on partners and families can be great, even when the individuals with HIV are well. Practical difficulties are seen particularly when individuals have severe illness or HIV-related brain disease. Significant levels of psychological distress are also common, including suicide ideation. Enhancing the self-esteem and coping skills of partners can help them to provide care for people with HIV. Living with HIV frequently impacts on relationships; communication may be difficult, sexual dysfunction may be experienced and the ways of coping adopted may not be advantageous to either partner. It can be beneficial to offer joint couple therapy. This support can often be provided by the mental health services attached to HIV care services. There are far fewer services available for parents and relatives of people with HIV disease. If local provision is not available, it can be useful to encourage parents to set up self-help groups.

References

BROWN, G.W. (1979) 'The social aetiology of depression – London studies', in Depue, R.A. (ed.) *The Psychobiology of the Depressive Disorders: Implications for the Effects of Stress*, San Diego CA: Academic Press.

BROWN, M.A. and POWELL-COPE, G. (1993) 'Themes of loss and dying for a family member with AIDS', *Research in Nursing and Health*, **16**, pp. 179–91.

BROWN, P.C. and SMITH, T.W. (1992) 'Social influence, marriage, and the heart: consequences of interpersonal control in husbands and wives', *Health Psychology*, **11**, pp. 88–96.

CARVER, C.S., SCHEIER, M.F. and WEINTRAUB, J.K. (1989) 'Assessing coping strategies: a theoretically based approach', *Journal of Personality and Social Psychology*, **56**, pp. 267–83.

CATALÁN, J., BURGESS, A. and KLIMES, I. (1995) *Psychological Medicine of HIV Infection*, Oxford: Oxford University Press.

CATALÁN, J., KLIMES, I., DAY, A., GARROD, A., BOND, A. and GALLWEY, J. (1992) 'The psychosocial impact of HIV infection in gay men – controlled investigation and factors associated with psychiatric morbidity', *British Journal of Psychiatry*, **161**, pp. 774–78.

CHESNEY, M.A., FOLKMAN, S. and CHAMBERS, D. (1996) 'Coping effectiveness training', *International Journal of STD and AIDS*, supplement 2, pp. 75–82.

COYLE, A. (1993) 'A study of psychological well being among gay men using the GHQ-30', *British Journal of Clinical Psychology*, **32**, pp. 218–20.

DEAN, L., HALL, W.E. and MARTIN, J.L. (1988) 'Chronic and intermittent AIDS related bereavement in a panel of homosexual men in New York City', *Journal of Palliative Care*, **4**, pp. 54–57.

DOKA, K.J. (1987) 'Silent sorrow: grief and the loss of significant others', *Death Studies*, **11**, pp. 455–69.

FOLEY, M., SKURNICK, J.H., KENNEDY, C.A., VALENTIN, R. and LOURIA, D.B. (1994) 'Family support for heterosexual partners in HIV-serodiscordant couples', *AIDS*, **8**, pp. 1483–87.

FOLKMAN, S. (1997) 'Positive psychological states and coping with severe stress', *Science and Medicine*, **45**, pp. 1207–21.

FOLKMAN, S., CHESNEY, M.A. and CHRISTOPHER-RICHARDS, A. (1994) 'Stress and coping in caregiving partners of men with AIDS', *Psychiatric Clinics of North America*, **17**, pp. 35–53.

FOLKMAN, S., CHESNEY, M.A., BOCCELLARI, A., COOKE, M. and COLLETTE, L. (1992) 'Death of a partner affects moods of HIV positive and HIV negative caregiving men differently', paper presented at the International Conference on AIDS, Amsterdam.

FOLKMAN, S., CHESNEY, M.A., COOKE, M., BOCCELLARI, A. and COLLETTE, L. (1994) 'Caregiver burden in HIV-positive and HIV-negative partners of men with AIDS', *Journal of Consulting and Clinical Psychology*, **62**, pp. 746–56.

FOLKMAN, S., CHESNEY, M.A., COLLETTE, L., BOCCELLARI, A. and COOKE, M. (1996) 'Post-bereavement depressive mood and its pre-bereavement predictors in HIV+ and HIV– partners of men with AIDS', *Journal of Personality and Social Psychology*, **70**, pp. 336–48.

GARDNER, W. and PREATOR, K. (1996) 'Children of seropositive mothers in the US AIDS epidemic', *Journal of Social Issues*, **52**, pp. 177–95.

GAZARIK, R. and FISCHMAN, D. (1995) 'A time-limited group for patients with HIV infection and their partners', *Group*, **19**, pp. 173–82.

GEORGE, H. (1990) 'Sexual and relationship problems among people affected by AIDS: three case studies', *Counselling Psychology Quarterly*, **3**, 389–99.

GILLEARD, C.J., BELFORD, H., GILLEARD, H., WHITTICK, J.E. and GLEDHILL, K. (1984) 'Emotional distress among the supporters of the elderly mentally infirm', *British Journal of Psychiatry*, **145**, pp. 172–77.

GREY, J. and HEDGE, B. (1999) 'Psychological distress and coping in the partners of gay men with HIV-related disease', *British Journal of Health Psychology*. In press.

HAYS, R.B., MAGEE, R.H. and CHAUNCEY, S. (1994) 'Identification of helpful and unhelpful behaviours of loved ones: the PWA's perspective', *AIDS Care*, **6**, pp. 379–92.

HEDGE, B. and GLOVER, L. (1990) 'Group intervention with HIV seropositive patients and their partners', *AIDS Care*, **2**, pp. 147–54.

IRVING, G., BOR, R. and CATALÁN, J. (1995) 'Psychological distress among gay men supporting a lover or partner with AIDS: a pilot study', *AIDS Care*, **7**, pp. 605–17.

KEMENY, M.E., WEINER, H., DURAN, R., TAYLOR, S.E. *et al.* (1995) 'Immune system changes after the death of a partner in HIV positive gay men', *Psychosomatic Medicine*, **57**, pp. 547–54.

KLIMES, I., CATALÁN, J., GARROD, A., DAY, A., BOND, A. and RIZZA, C. (1992) 'Partners of men with HIV infection and haemophilia: controlled investigation and factors associated with psychological morbidity', *AIDS Care*, **4**, pp. 149–56.

LAURICHESSE, H.A., MORTIMER, J., EVANS, B.G. and FARRINGTON, C.P. (1998) 'Pre-AIDS mortality in HIV-infected individuals in England, Wales and Northern Ireland, 1982–1996', *AIDS*, **12**, pp. 651–58.

LENNON, M.C., MARTIN, J.L. and DEAN, L. (1990) 'The influence of social support on AIDS related grief reactions among gay men', *Social Science and Medicine*, **31**, pp. 477–84.

LYNN, L.A. and SILVERMAN, J.J. (1996) 'A comparison of HIV positive and HIV negative caregivers of patients with HIV infection', paper presented at the Eleventh International AIDS Conference, Vancouver.

McCANN, K. and WADSWORTH, E. (1992) 'The role of informal carers in supporting gay men who have HIV related disease: what do they do and what are their needs?' *AIDS Care*, **4**, pp. 25–34.

McGINN, F. (1996) 'The plight of rural parents caring for an adult child with HIV', *Families in Society*, **77**, pp. 269–78.

McKUSICK, L. (1991) 'Multiple loss accounts for worsening distress in a community heavily hit by AIDS', paper presented at the Seventh International Conference on AIDS, Florence.

MARTIN, J.L.M. (1998) 'Psychological consequences of AIDS-related bereavement among gay men', *Journal of Consulting and Clinical Psychology*, **36**, pp. 856–62.

MARTIN, J.L. and DEAN, L. (1993) 'Effects of AIDS-related bereavement among gay men: a 7-year longitudinal study 1985–1991', *Journal of Consulting and Clinical Psychology*, **61**, pp. 94–103.

MIDDLETON, W., RAPHAEL, B., BURNETT, P. and MARTINEK, N. (1997) 'Psychological distress and bereavement', *Journal of Nervous and Mental Disease*, **185**, pp. 447–53.

MORRIS, L.W., MORRIS, R.G. and BRITTON, P.G. (1988) 'The relationship between marital intimacy, perceived strain and depression in spouse caregivers of dementia sufferers', *British Journal of Medical Psychology*, **61**, pp. 231–36.

MOSKOWITZ, J.-T., FOLKMAN, S., COLLETTE, L. and VITTINGHOFF, E. (1996) 'Coping and mood during AIDS-related bereavement', *Annals of Behavioural Medicine*, **18**, pp. 49–57.

OSTROW, D.G., GRANT, I. and ATKINSON, J.H. (1988) 'Assessment and management of the AIDS patient with neuropsychiatric disturbance', *Journal of Clinical Psychiatry*, **49**, pp. 14–22.

OSTROW, D.G., JOSEPH, J., MONJAN, A., KESSLER, R., EMMONS, C., PHAIR, J., FOX, R., KINGSLEY, L., DUDLEY, J., CHMEIL, J.S. and VAN RADEN, M. (1986) 'Psychosocial aspects of AIDS risk', *Psychopharmacological Bulletin*, **22**, pp. 678–83.

PAKENHAM, K.I., DADDS, M.R. and TERRY, D.J. (1994) 'Relationship between adjustment to HIV and both social support and coping', *Journal of Consulting and Clinical Psychology*, **62**, pp. 1194–1203.

PAKENHAM, K.I., DADDS, M.R. and TERRY, D.J. (1995) 'Carers' burden and adjustment to HIV', *AIDS Care*, **7**, pp. 189–203.

PALELLA, F.J., DELANEY, K.M., MOORMAN, A.C. *et al.* (1998) 'Declining morbidity and mortality among patients with advanced human immunodeficiency virus infection', *New England Journal of Medicine*, **338**, pp. 853–60.

PAYKEL, E.S., PRUSOFF, B.A. and MYERS, J.K. (1975) 'Suicide attempts and recent life events', *Archives of General Psychiatry*, **32**, pp. 327–33.

PERAKYLA, A. and BOR, R. (1990) 'Interactional problems of addressing "dreaded issues" in HIV-counselling', *AIDS Care*, **2**, pp. 325–38.

PINCHING, A.J. (1994) 'AIDS: health care ethics and society', in Gillon, R. (ed.) *Principles of Health Care Ethics*, Chichester: Wiley.

POWELL-COPE, G. (1995) 'The experiences of gay couples affected by HIV infection', *Qualitative Health Research*, **5**, pp. 36–62.

RABINS, P.V., FITTING, M.D., EASTHAM, J. and FETTING, J. (1990) 'The emotional impact of caring for the chronically ill', *Psychosomatics*, **31**, pp. 331–36.

RAVEIS, V.H. and SIEGEL, K. (1991) 'The impact of caregiving on informal or familial caregivers', *AIDS Patient Care*, **5**, pp. 39–43.

RICHMOND, B.J. and ROSS, M. (1994) 'Responses to AIDS related bereavement', *Journal of Psychosocial Oncology*, **12**, pp. 143–63.

ROSENGARD, C. and FOLKMAN, S. (1997) 'Suicide ideation, bereavement, HIV serostatus and psychological variables in partners of men with AIDS', *AIDS Care*, **9**, pp. 373–84.

SCHNEIDER, S.G., TAYLOR, S.E., KEMENY, M.E. and DUDLEY, J. (1991) 'Factors influencing suicide intent in gay and bisexual suicide ideators: differing models for men with and without human immunodeficiency virus', *Journal of Personality and Social Psychology*, **61**, pp. 776–88.

SCHWARTZBERG, S. (1992) 'AIDS-related bereavement among gay men:

the inadequacy of current theories of grief', *Psychotherapy*, **29**, pp. 422–29.

SLATER, J. and DEPUE, R.A. (1981) 'The contribution of environmental events and social support to serious suicide attempts in primary depressive disorder', *Journal of Abnormal Psychology*, **90**, pp. 275–85.

STEMPLE, R.R., MOULTON, J.M. and MOSS, A.R. (1995) 'Self-disclosure of HIV-1 antibody test results: The San Francisco General Hospital cohort', *AIDS Education and Prevention*, **7**, pp. 116–23.

STROEBE, M.S. and STROEBE, W. (1983) 'Who suffers more? Sex differences in health risks of the widowed', *Psychological Bulletin*, **93**, pp. 279–301.

TURNER, H.A. and CATANIA, J.A. (1997) 'Informal caregiving to persons with AIDS in the United States: caregiver burden among central cities residents eighteen to forty-nine years old', *American Journal of Community Psychology*, **25**, pp. 35–59.

USSHER, J. (1990) 'Cognitive behavioural couples therapy with gay men referred for counselling in an AIDS setting: a pilot study', *AIDS Care*, **2**, pp. 43–51.

WACHOLDER, R. (1993) 'Carers and spinal cord injury: emotional impact and psychosocial moderating factors', unpublished dissertation, copies at British Psychological Society and Oxford in-service training course in clinical psychology.

WOODS, R.T. and BRITTON, P.G. (1985) *Clinical Psychology with the elderly*, London: Croom-Helm.

WRUBEL, J. and FOLKMAN, S. (1997) 'What informal caregivers actually do: the caregiving skills of partners of men with AIDS', *AIDS Care*, **9**, pp. 691–706.

Chapter 5

Dementia Associated with HIV Infection

Edwina Williams

This chapter offers a detailed exploration of HIV dementia. Having explained the three major classification systems, it considers the epidemiology: how differences in diagnosis affect estimates of prevalence and incidence. This section also examines the risk factors. Then follow sections on prognosis, the clinical features of HIV dementia, differential diagnosis, and how the disease develops. Investigation and disease management are next. Finally, it looks at prevention and considers possibilities for the future.

Introduction

Snider was the first to recognize and report that HIV infection affected the central nervous system (Snider *et al.*, 1983). Shortly after this a syndrome of dementia was described in people with advanced HIV infection (Navia, Jordan and Price, 1986; Navia *et al.*, 1986). This was followed by reports of cognitive deficits in asymptomatic individuals with HIV infection (Grant *et al.*, 1987). There was, initially, concern that the onset of cognitive impairment occurred early in the infection, and there were fears that the dementia was far more common than now appears to be the case. The dementia associated with HIV has been known as AIDS dementia complex (ADC), sub-acute encephalitis, HIV encephalopathy, HIV-1 associated cognitive motor complex and most recently HIV-1 associated dementia. These terms are not strictly interchangeable but have often been used that way. It is therefore not surprising that they have often caused misunderstanding. This confusion in terminology initially made the interpretation of research difficult. More recently, the careful observations of clinicians and development of carefully defined diagnostic criteria has enabled researchers to form conclusions about many issues relating to the HIV dementia.

The multicentre AIDS cohort study (MACS) into the neuropsychological consequences of HIV infection illustrates this new and precise research. Its long-term follow-up of a group of HIV-infected individuals over nine years disproved initial concerns that asymptomatic individuals showed significant cognitive decline (Sacktor *et al.*, 1996). The dementia syndrome has a high morbidity and mortality and is predominantly a generalized central nervous system disorder with preserved consciousness (Price, 1996). The mechanisms through which HIV causes central nervous system disorders are not fully understood; there are two principal ways whereby these disorders occur. Primary disorders like the dementia syndrome are the result of the direct effects of HIV on nervous tissue, and secondary disorders are caused by opportunistic infections, tumours and other conditions secondary to immune dysfunction and systemic manifestations of the disease.

Concepts and Definitions

Accurate diagnosis is paramount, as anyone suffering from AIDS may have cerebral complications which can potentially confound the clinician. Accurate diagnosis enables the dementia to be recognized and managed clinically in individual patients; it is also crucial for research. Lack of precision in diagnosis may have far-reaching effects on research evaluation. The newer classification systems tend to fine-tune earlier ones. Ensuring strict diagnosis develops a better understanding of the syndrome, hence the symptoms and signs that may be seen, and this in turn guides the appropriate investigation of the patient. There are three different ways in which the dementia syndrome in HIV is defined

AIDS Dementia Complex

The first detailed description of AIDS dementia complex (ADC) came from a retrospective clinical and neuropathological study (Navia, Jordan and Price, 1986; Navia *et al.*, 1986). The clinical description of cognitive and behavioural changes consisted of a triad of symptoms and signs: cognitive impairment, motor dysfunction and behavioural changes. The problem with this concept was that it assumed the three features always occurred together. This meant the diagnosis of ADC could be made even if the three features were not present, and it therefore became possible to have a diagnosis of dementia without, for example, memory impairment.

Further refinement was provided by the development of a clinical rating scale (Price and Brew, 1988). It has been widely used in research. It has six stages: 0=no ADC; 0.5 and 1=mild ADC; 2, 3 and 4=more severe ADC. Mild ADC means there is difficulty with concentration and mental agility (list making and rereading are required and individuals may forget what they are saying). The motor abnormalities are subclinical (slowing of rapid movement of the extremities and eyes). In more severe ADC the cognitive impairment chiefly results in psychomotor retardation (slowing of the thought processes). A wider cognitive impairment also occurs. There are diffuse motor abnormalities with release reflexes on neurological testing (such as the snout response). The motor impairment may be so severe that quadriparesis occurs. Vacuolar myelopathy affecting the spinal cord (Dal Pan, Glass and McArthur, 1994) was also considered part of ADC. In this type of ADC an early complication is a spastic ataxic gait which causes difficulty walking. There are also hyperactive deep tendon reflexes found on physical examination. The ADC clinical rating scale has been criticized as being imprecise and with questionable validity and reliability (Everall, 1995). A further problem is that mild degrees of cognitive, motor and behavioural dysfunction may lead to a diagnosis ADC whereas other definitions of dementia would require substantial cognitive impairment. If the concept of ADC is to be used, it is important to be aware that a diagnosis of ADC, especially in its mild form, does not necessarily mean that someone has dementia in the usual sense of the word.

HIV-1 Associated Dementia

HIV-1 associated dementia is the formal title from the Tenth International Classification of Diseases (ICD10) developed in 1990 (World Health Organization, 1990). It has operationally defined criteria, which means the diagnostic categories are scientifically developed and tested. These are derived from those of dementia in ICD10. To receive the diagnosis it is necessary to have objectively verified decline in memory and intellectual ability with evidence of HIV-1 infection and the symptoms must have been present for at least one month. There must also be an absence of other causes of a similar clinical profile or impaired consciousness (delirium). Unlike with many other dementias, it is uncommon to find aphasia, agnosia and apraxia (disorders of the brain affecting language, sensation and skilled movement respectively). HIV-1 dementia is compatible with other ICD10 dementias. The criteria are more useful and detailed and they are comparable to pre-existing systems such as DSM IV. The diagnosis is further divided into mild, moderate and severe categories. This classificatory system and the DSM IV system have realigned AIDS dementia with other dementias.

HIV-1 Associated Cognitive Motor Complex

The American Academy of Neurology (AAN) has also set up diagnostic criteria (American Academy of Neurology AIDS Task Force, 1991). 'HIV-1 associated cognitive motor complex' is the name of this diagnostic category and it is consistent with the WHO definition. It is subdivided into different variants of the disease. 'HIV-1 associated myelopathy' is the subtype where there is primarily motor impairment. There is also 'HIV-1 associated dementia complex' where there is primarily cognitive impairment (memory problems and intellectual decline). There is also a list of criteria for possible or probable diagnosis. It may be subdivided further and they suggest the category 'HIV-1 associated minor cognitive/motor disorder'. Ultimately, the AAN and WHO criteria both describe a subcortical dementia characterized by slowness and imprecision in cognitive and motor control (Anon, 1990).

Epidemiology

In view of the problems with definition, classification and diagnosis described above, epidemiological estimates have varied widely, and only recently has the picture become clear. A number of factors may affect estimates; for example, criteria for diagnosis vary widely, particularly the severity threshold of the dementia. Another important factor has been the means of obtaining subjects for study; for example, subjects may be selected because of their neurological disease from specialist neurology clinics. This may lead to a preponderance of neurological symptoms in descriptions of the clinical picture. Dementia is known to develop mainly in patients with late HIV and severe immuno-suppression, therefore prevalence differs according to stage of infection, i.e. the degree of immunosuppression, in the group studied (McArthur *et al.*, 1993; Bacellar *et al.*, 1994). Changes in the HIV disease process may also have affected the results of investigations. There may have been spontaneous changes in the virus or treatment of HIV which may have changed the course of the disease. Epidemiological investigations have typically been in Western gay men, so more studies are necessary in different populations; the preva-lence found may also differ between developed and developing countries.

Prevalence and Incidence

Prevalence is the percentage of the population with the disease at a specific point in time. Early studies quote a range of prevalence figures from 16% to 38%. All these studies used broad criteria for diagnosis and included selected groups of individuals, such as patients from neurology clinics (Navia, Jordan and Price, 1986; Navia *et al.*, 1986; McArthur, 1987; De Gans and Portegies *et al.*, 1989). One study which showed a prevalence rate of 54% may be consid-ered anomalous, as a very low threshold for dementia was used (Howlett *et al.*, 1989). More recent studies have shown much lower figures than these. A study using AAN criteria found a dementia prevalence of 6% (McArthur *et al.*, 1993).

Most studies have focused on developed countries but there appears to be little variation in the prevalence of HIV dementia around the world (Belec *et al.*, 1989; Perriens *et al.*, 1992). This has been demonstrated most convincingly by the WHO Multicenter Cross-cultural Organization in a study of ambula-tory patients from five centres in 1990. This is perhaps the most accurate study to date because of the use of ICD10 diagnostic criteria. The prevalence ranged from 0% in Thailand to 6.9% in Kenya. The very low percentage found in Thailand was probably due to the disease reaching the country shortly before the study period. This suggests that the length of infection is an important factor in the development of dementia because in the rest of the countries studied the range was 5.4–6.9%. The study was confined to outpatients only, which makes it likely that more severely ill patients with dementia were not included. The prevalence of dementia is therefore likely to be somewhat higher (Maj, Janssen and Satz, 1991; Maj *et al.*, 1994a,b). Although many investigations into the prevalence of HIV dementia have used different criteria, they have consistently found it to be present in less than 10% of people with AIDS.

Incidence is the rate of development of a disease over a period of time. Estimates have only started to emerge as data is accumulating. The incidence of HIV dementia did not change significantly between 1988 and 1992, when definite and probable cases were examined by MACS (Bacellar *et al.*, 1994). It was found to be 1.76 per 100 person years. Person years are the total number of years free of the specific disease – in this case HIV dementia.

Risk Factors

A number of factors are known to influence the prevalence of dementia. The first of these is the increased risk of developing dementia as the CD4 count falls; this is especially the case when the CD4 count falls below 200. Table 5.1 illustrates the results of the MACS study; it shows the incidence over a five-year period (Bacellar *et al.*, 1994). The development of dementia is more likely at the extremes of age. The risk increases with increased age (McArthur *et al.*, 1993; Baldeweg, Catalán and Gazzard, 1998) and children infected by vertical transmission or perinatally are also particularly vulnerable. (Epstein *et al.*, 1986; Belman *et al.*, 1985; Diamond *et al.*, 1987). A recent, large study of 1,500 patients found no differences in incidence between risk groups (Baldeweg, Catalán and Gazzard, 1998). It was previously thought that people infected by intravenous drug use were more likely to develop dementia than those infected via other routes. One study found that the risk may be 50% greater

Table 5.1 *Results of the MACS study*

CD4 count (cells/mm³)	Incidence per 100 person years
<100	7.34
101–200	3.04
201–350	1.31
351–500	1.75
>500	0.46

Source: Bacellar *et al.* (1994).

(Chiesi *et al.*, 1996) but this is likely to have been influenced by the finding that injecting drug users have higher rates of cognitive impairment regardless of their serostatus (Egan *et al.*, 1990). There is also some evidence that women develop dementia more frequently than men (Chiesi *et al.*, 1996); this too has been contradicted (Baldeweg, Catalán and Gazzard, 1998). Low haemoglobin appears to be associated with an increased risk of developing dementia (Baldeweg, Catalán and Gazzard, 1998; McArthur *et al.*, 1993) Low body mass index was also thought to entail a greater risk (McArthur *et al.*, 1993). The presence of more constitutional symptoms may also be associated with an increased risk of dementia (McArthur *et al.*, 1993).

Although substantial neurological impairment has been reported in a few asymptomatic individuals (Grant *et al.*, 1987), most investigators agree that severe impairment is rare in early infection if other factors such as education, age and substance abuse are taken into account (Selnes *et al.*, 1992; van Gorp *et al.*, 1994).

Prognosis

The onset and progression of HIV dementia varies widely. It usually occurs late in HIV infection when the CD4 count falls below 200. The neurological deficits that are associated with dementia usually develop insidiously, though occasionally they may develop rapidly. When HIV dementia presents, the prognosis is generally poor (Selnes *et al.*, 1991). It is known that there is a shorter survival in patients with HIV dementia compared with people who are HIV positive and who have comparable degrees of dysfunction without any cognitive impairment (Mayeux *et al.*, 1993). Early reports stated that 50% of individuals with ADC developed a severe form of the disorder within 2 months and there was a mean survival of approximately 4 months; however, 20% had a lengthy course (Navia, Jordan and Price, 1986; Navia *et al.*, 1986). The MACS study has reported a median life expectancy of 6 months (McArthur *et al.*, 1993). However, this data includes information collected before the introduction of HAART – the new highly active antiretroviral therapies, otherwise known as combination therapies. It is expected that new treatments will have a favourable effect on the prognosis of HIV associated dementia.

Clinical Features

In advanced HIV dementia, self-report of cognitive impairment reflects cognitive performance on psychometric testing accurately; however, this is often the case early in HIV dementia even though the changes on testing may be subtle.

The dementia presents with predominantly subcortical features (Navia, 1990) and displays the following clinical picture. The cognitive impairment is manifest as forgetfulness, decreased concentration, confusion and slowness of thought. The profound amnesia typical of other dementias, such as Alzheimer's disease, occasionally occurs in the later stages but is not a common finding. The motor problems exhibit as slowing with loss of balance and poor coordination, leg weakening and deterioration in handwriting. The behavioural changes are seen as apathy and social withdrawal; regression may be an aspect of the picture. The cortical signs of apraxia, agnosia and aphasia generally indicate that other pathological processes are occurring. Organic psychoses, such as mania, have been reported as being the first manifestation of HIV dementia, but the significance of this is uncertain (Lyketsos *et al.*, 1993, 1997).

As the dementia advances, the cognitive decline becomes more marked, as do the psychomotor retardation and behavioural abnormalities. Objective neurological signs also become more apparent, usually in the form of paraparesis, incontinence, tremor and seizures. Neuropsychiatric tests may be useful to detect early cognitive dysfunction and are used to chart the course and progression of the disease (Sidtis *et al.*, 1988; Tross *et al.*, 1988; Derix *et al.*, 1990).

Differential Diagnosis

The diagnosis of HIV associated dementia is, to some extent, reached by exclusion. It requires positive evidence for memory impairment and intellectual decline, but besides that it is essential to exclude other possible causes of cognitive impairment. The neurological complications of HIV are closely related to the degree of immunosuppression which is measured by the CD4 count. This helps to predict what other diseases may affect the central nervous system when forming the differential diagnosis. Other diseases may mimic or coexist with the dementia. This is especially important in the severely immunocompromised patient as the likelihood of multiple pathology is high. The problems can be grouped in the following manner. The first group are focal lesions (areas of tissue which are damaged, resulting in impaired function) of the central nervous system, producing space-occupying lesions which interfere with brain function. The most common causes are cerebral toxoplasmosis, lymphoma of the central nervous system and progressive multifocal leukoencephalopathy. The second group are caused by other opportunistic infections. Here the infection affects the brain tissue more uniformly; examples are cytomegalovirus, cryptococcal meningitis and neurosyphilis.

Another problem, delirium, may be caused by any severe illness from metabolic disturbance to infection, or it may be related to prescribed medication. The underlying cause of the delirium in this instance does not have to be related to the brain directly and may be found anywhere in the body. Finally, depression must be considered and excluded. This is particularly important in the early stages of the dementia where the behaviour change may be slight. In depression, patients often complain of memory impairment. It is important to note that this particular complaint of memory problems is related to poor concentration and loss of interest. When memory is formally tested in depression, true impairment is not elicited.

Table 5.2 illustrates the symptoms that people frequently complain of when they present to their doctors. It is not exhaustive nor is it absolute, as there may be instances when the symptoms are not present or when other symptoms are present instead. It is intended to demonstrate the overlap in the presentations of different problems; this shows the difficulty in making an accurate diagnosis without the assistance of investigations. Table 5.3 illustrates the findings on examination. It too demonstrates the overlap between HIV dementia and other problems that may cause memory impairment.

Aetiology

Aetiology is a rapidly changing area, so this section aims to provide the reader with an overview of the situation. A number of factors contribute to the development of dementia. The immune system suppresses viral replication until late in infection; however, immunosuppression is not the only factor in determining the development of HIV dementia, because not all those who are HIV positive develop HIV dementia. There are many abnormal findings in the brains of individuals who have suffered from HIV dementia.

HIV Infection in the Brain

HIV enters the central nervous system soon after infection (McArthur *et al.*, 1988; Goulsmith *et al.*, 1996; Ho *et al.*, 1985; Davis *et al.*, 1992), possibly inside infected peripheral monocytes (Peluso *et al.*, 1985) or by infected T cells passing through the damaged blood – brain barrier (Michaels, Sharer and Epstein, 1988). The virus remains latent in the brain for many years, although some minor non-specific neuropathological abnormalities may be seen in people with asymptomatic infection (Lenhardt, Super and Wiley, 1988; Lantos *et al.*, 1989; Esiri *et al.*, 1990; Gray *et al.*, 1992). Major neuropathological abnormalities become increasingly common as the HIV progresses. At least 80% of people who die with AIDS will have some HIV-related neuropathology; frequently this is opportunistic infection, lymphoma or cerebrovascular lesions (Petito *et al.*, 1986; Budka *et al.*, 1987; Lantos *et al.*, 1989). Individuals who have died of AIDS typically have 30–50% fewer cortical neurones than age-matched and sex-matched controls (Everall, Luthert and Lantos, 1993).

HIV-infected cells are mainly found in the white matter of the brain. They are mostly of the monocyte–macrophage series but are sometimes infected endothelial cells (Wiley, Masliah and Morey, 1991). HIV has been identified in

Table 5.2 *Symptoms of presentation*

Problem[a]	CD4 count	Memory loss	Behaviour change	Gait disturbance	Headache	Fever	Delirium	Neck stiffness	Weakness	Lethargy or apathy	Seizures	Visual disturbance
HIV dementia	<200	−	−	+								
TE	<200				+	+	+				+	
CNM	<200	−			+	+	+	+		+		
CNS lymphoma	<100	−			+		+			+	+	
PML	<100						+		+	+		−
CMV encephalitis	<50						+		+	+		
Neurosyphilis	any	−			+			+				−
Depression	any	−	−							+		

[a] *Key to abbreviation:* TE = toxoplasma encephalitis, CNM = *Cryptococcus neoformans* meningitis, PML = progressive multifocal leukoencephalopathy. *Source:* Simpson and Tagliati (1994).

Table 5.3 *Signs found on examination*

Problem[a]	Dementia	Spasticity	Ataxia	Hemiparesis	Aphasia	Cranial nerve palsies
HIV dementia	–	+				
Toxoplasma encephalitis	–		+	+		
CNM						+
CNS lymphoma	–			+	+	
PML			+	+		
CMV encephalitis	–	+				+
Neurosyphilis	–					+
Depression						

[a] *Key to abbreviations*: CNM = *Cryptococcus neoformans* meningitis, PML = progressive multifocal leukoencephalopathy.
Source: Simpson and Tagliati (1994).

the brains of patients with HIV dementia by using Southern blot techniques, in situ hybridization (Shaw *et al.*, 1985) and polymerase chain reaction (Pang *et al.*, 1990). These techniques which examine DNA have also shown infection in a wider range of cells such as astrocytes, vascular endothelial cells and neurones (Dickson *et al.*, 1994) but the importance of the infection of these cells is uncertain.

The virus affects the brain directly, most commonly, causing HIV encephalitis and HIV leukoencephalopathy (Ketlzer *et al.*, 1990; Everall, Luthert and Lantos, 1991, 1993; Wiley, Masliah and Morey, 1991). The requirements for a diagnosis of HIV encephalitis are the presence of the inflammatory cells – microglia, macrophages, multinucleate giant cells – and the presence of HIV-infected cells in the central nervous system (Budka *et al.*, 1991). They are found throughout the white matter of the basal ganglia, brain stem and cortex. However, the pathological changes seen in the brain may not be as marked as the clinical symptoms seen in life. The amount of virus present in the brain does not relate to the severity of the histopathological features (Boni *et al.*, 1993). The ability of the virus to reproduce well in macrophages and microglia in the brain but poorly in lymphocyte-derived cells elsewhere in the body is known as macrophage tropism (O'Brien, 1994). New genetic strains of HIV have emerged which have increased macrophage tropism. Macrophage tropism causes macrophages and microglial cells to fuse (Dickson *et al.*, 1994), forming multinucleated cells characteristic of encephalitis. HIV leukoencephalopathy is a technical term for diffuse white matter pallor (Navia *et al.*, 1986). It is thought to be caused by demyelination and astrocytosis in the white matter of cerebral hemispheres and cerebellum. Some authors believe there is no evidence of primary demyelination, leading them to conclude that the alteration in the blood–brain barrier contributes to the development of HIV dementia (Power *et al.*, 1993).

Regardless of whether there is HIV encephalitis, there is an increase in the concentration of serum proteins in the brain with HIV infection – evidence of damage to the blood–brain barrier (Pettito *et al.*, 1986). These serum proteins are found in the subcortical white matter glia and the frontal cortical neurones (Power *et al.*, 1993). Although multinucleated giant cells and diffuse myelin pallor are found only in those with a clinical history of dementia, not all those with dementia show either of these signs (Glass *et al.*, 1993).

Toxic Mechanisms

Cells derived from the neuroectoderm – neurones and oligodendrocytes – are damaged despite being largely uninfected, and there is neuronal loss in patients with HIV encephalopathy (Ketzler *et al.*, 1990; Everall, Luthert and Lantos, 1991). Cell-to-cell interaction between HIV-infected monocytes and HIV-infected astrocytes amplifies effects of HIV infection, leading to neurotoxic factors and glial proliferation (Epstein and Gendelman, 1993). It may be that macrophage and microglial infection cause neurotoxic substances to develop. The first of these toxic substances are gene products. When HIV infects astrocytes the viral gene produces a number of surface glycoproteins, particularly gp120 and the regulatory gene products *tat* and *nef*. In cell culture experiments these substances lead to neuronal death causing calcium channels to open in neuronal membranes (Dreyer *et al.*, 1990). The calcium channel blocking drug, nimodipine, prevents this neuronal death in cell cultures and the damage caused by gp120 is blocked by the *N*-methyl-D aspartate antagonist nemantidine (Lipton *et al.*, 1991). Glutamate depletion supports this hypothesis (Grimaldi *et al.*, 1991; Cvetkovitch *et al.*, 1992).

Cytokines are produced in many neurodegenerative diseases and HIV dementia is no exception (Choi, 1988). Cytokine pathways activate *N*-methyl-D-aspartate receptors and encourage nitric oxide production (Price, 1996); both substances are neurotoxic. Cytokines such as tumour necrosis factor α and interleukin-6 – metabolites of the arachidonic acid cascade – are produced by feedback mechanisms (Epstein and Gendelman, 1993; Genis *et al.*, 1992) High levels of tumour necrosis factor are proportional to the cognitive impairment and neurone damage that occurs. (Glass *et al.*, 1993; Wesselingh *et al.*, 1993). It may be that cytokine-mediated alteration of the blood–brain barrier leads to viral entry into the brain (Simpson and Tagliati, 1994). Quinolinic acid is an excitotoxin which is an *N*-methyl-D aspartate agonist. Investigations have shown that this substance is increased (Heyes *et al.*, 1989, 1990, 1991) leading to increased cytokine production.

Microglobulins and neopterin are markers of immune activation. β_2-microglobulin is a low molecular weight protein (McArthur *et al.*, 1992) present on the surface of cells such as lymphocytes and macrophages. It is increased in the cerebrospinal fluid in HIV dementia. The levels of β_2-microglobulin (Brew *et al.*, 1989) and neopterin (Brew *et al.*, 1990) in cerebrospinal fluid arc proportional to the severity of dementia. HIV gp41 antigen was found in brains using immunohistochemical techniques. The gp41 immune reactivity was proportional to loss of neocortical dendritic area and synapses (Masliah *et al.*, 1992).

Investigations

The diagnosis of HIV associated dementia is made by a process of exclusion and is supported by neuroimaging (Aylward *et al.*, 1993) and, most importantly, psychometric studies (Seilhean *et al.*, 1993). Investigations should be commenced only after a careful history and physical examination have been completed. The diagnosis relies ultimately upon clinical judgement according to operationalized criteria. Certain tests are, however, necessary to confirm the diagnosis and exclude other pathologies.

The main importance of blood screening and cerebral spinal fluid is to exclude other pathologies. This involves searching for systemic infections which may present with a picture similar to dementia – such as VDRL tests, for syphilis; cryptococcal antigen and the presence of JC virus (Jesus Christ virus) which is linked to PML (progressive multifocal leukoencephalopathy). Cerebrospinal fluid abnormalities are frequently found in HIV dementia, but findings are inconsistent. Lymphocytes may be increased. There may be increased protein caused by an increase in the total immunoglobulin fraction because of the intrathecal synthesis of anti HIV IgG. However, these changes are frequently found with HIV infection without neurological symptoms (McArthur *et al.*, 1988). Substances which act as markers of immune activation such as β_2-microglobulin, neopterin and quinolinate may also support the diagnosis (Meillet *et al.*, 1993; Heyes *et al.*, 1991; McArthur *et al.*, 1992; Brew *et al.*, 1989, 1990) these too may be found in opportunistic infection and lymphoma of the central nervous system.

Neuroradiology is an important part of the assessment. CT (computed tomography) and MRI (magnetic resonance imaging) scans are used to exclude infection and neoplasm and support the diagnosis because of changes of cerebral atrophy, ventricular enlargement and diffuse multifocal white matter abnormalities also present in the basal ganglia (Navia *et al.*, 1986; Post *et al.*, 1988; Olsen *et al.*, 1988). The amount of atrophy is related to the severity of the dementia (Dal Pan *et al.*, 1992; Aylward *et al.*, 1993), though this is controversial (Portegies *et al.*, 1993). The cerebral atrophy leads to enlarged lateral ventricles and cerebrospinal fluid space within the expanded cerebral sulci. None of the tests discussed so far are sufficiently reliable or specific to make the diagnosis alone.

Once the investigations are completed to exclude other pathologies, cognitive function may be assessed. The neuropsychology of healthy populations is extensive, which allows accurate assessment of impaired cognitive function. It involves tests of memory and verbal fluency, for example. The tests localize deficits to anatomical sites in the brain. The pattern of deficits is very characteristic for HIV dementia. This makes neuropsychology the most useful assessment as it confirms diagnosis. The assessment may be refined for HIV dementia by concentrating on assessment of psychomotor speed and memory (Butters *et al.*, 1990; Burgess and Thornton, 1995).

Psychophysiology includes electroencephalography (EEG), multimodal evoked potentials (MEP) and event-related potentials (ERP). They all involve measuring the electrical activity of the brain. These tests are very sensitive to changes in brain function (Harden *et al.*, 1993; Parisi, Strosselli and Di Perri, 1988); however, they are not sufficiently specific to be clinically useful, because the traces do not show a characteristic pattern seen only in HIV dementia. Electrophysiology has not been widely performed on people without health problems, which limits its uses in clinical assessment; it is mainly used for research. Occasionally, it is useful for long-term assessment by comparing traces from first presentation with those at a later date.

Management

Medication

Drug Treatments of HIV and Adjuvant Therapies

There has been a great deal of progress in the field of drug treatments, but few medications have been demonstrated to be specifically effective for HIV dementia. The only established one is zidovudine (AZT). The risk of developing dementia is significantly lower when people have taken zidovudine (Baldeweg, Catalán and Gazzard, 1998; Chiesi *et al.*, 1996). Treatment with this drug for at least 6 months is necessary to provide protection, though long-term treatment of greater than 18 months has not been found beneficial (Baldeweg, Catalán and Gazzard, 1998). Many new drugs are being developed but efficacy is yet to be established. Zidovudine enters the brain in higher concentrations than most other antiretrovirals, which may account for its efficacy. Very recent research has demonstrated, in a small group of individuals, that when lamivudine is combined with either stavudine or zidovudine both drug combinations were equally effective in reducing HIV-1 RNA concentrations in the cerebrospinal fluid (Foudraine et al., 1998). It is interesting that the concentration of the drugs in the blood stream was unrelated to the concentration of the drugs in the cerebrospinal fluid but the importance of this finding lies in the fact that antiretroviral drugs other than zidovudine might be useful in the prevention of HIV dementia. It is certain that this will be followed by further research.

There is a significant problem when drugs are developed, because most clinical trials do not evaluate neuropsychological function and how the new drug affects this. Once approved for clinical use, it is difficult to find an ethical justification for randomized controlled trials of the treatment in relation to cognitive impairment.

HIV infection does lead to brain injury, so antiretroviral measures are effective. It is essential that they are able to enter the brain. As there are downstream toxic pathways, this provides the possibility of adjuvant therapies by non-antiretroviral drugs. A number of other drugs have been assessed in clinical trials: neuroprotective drugs acting on primary target cells and compensatory drugs acting on neural networks (Price, 1995). These include nimodipine, a calcium channel blocker; pentoxyphylline, a tumour necrosis factor antagonist; nemantidine, an N-methyl-D-aspartate antagonist; and peptide T, a pentapeptide analogue of gp120 (Pert *et al.*, 1988).

Drug Treatments of Related Disorders

Psychostimulants such as methylphenedate and dextroamphetamine have been used as treatment for low mood and cognitive impairment often seen with HIV dementia. There may be unpleasant side effects, such as agitation, anorexia and difficulties managing elevated mood, so they require careful application and monitoring. There is also a risk of misuse (Fernandez and Levy, 1990). The use of sedatives or antipsychotic medication in mood disorders has also been used (Lyketsos *et al.*, 1993, 1997).

HIV dementia may be associated with delirium; the antipsychotic drug haloperidol has been used in this situation (Ostrow, Grant and Atkinson, 1988; Breitbart *et al.*, 1996). There is a risk of extrapyramidal side effects with haloperidol (Hriso *et al.*, 1991). More recent work has suggested the use of atypical antipsychotic drugs which are less likely to cause these unpleasant problems because of their low striatal action (Scurlock, Singh and Catalán, 1995; Singh and Catalán, 1994). These drugs may also help with the behavioural problems associated with HIV dementia (Catalán, Burgess and Klimes, 1995).

Psychological Therapies

The early reports of high risk of developing dementia with HIV led to a great deal of fear. Research then confirmed that it was important to discuss the diagnosis clearly and sensitively, and this is still the case (Green and Kocsis, 1988; Kocsis, 1989). Behavioural problems and mood disorders need to be recognized and treated appropriately; however, there may be a role for more active psychotherapies which focus on assisting the individual to come to terms with their loss of mental powers and independence. Discussion may also cover issues such as legal matters, financial decisions and provision of care as well as advanced directives to doctors. Partners, caregivers and relatives are at high risk of developing psychological disorders; counselling has therefore been suggested to provide for these problems (Meadows and Catalán, 1994).

Social Interventions

Adequate nursing and social support are vital if the person with HIV dementia is to remain at home. If behavioural disturbance becomes profound, psychiatric care may be required (Ostrow, Harris and Mill, 1992; Esterson, Harris and Kessinger, 1992). This situation may arise if the dementia is so severe that it is no longer possible to live at home with support from friends, relatives and professional carers. It may be due to increased nursing requirements or behavioural disturbance. At this point the individual may need respite care or residential care (Sims and Moss, 1991; Cantacuzino, 1994; Florence, 1994; Meadows and Catalán, 1994). Respite care is when periods of time are spent in residential facilities to allow carers to rest. It allows them to continue looking after the person suffering from dementia. Long-term residential care entails nursing care in a specialist unit which can provide the facilities required to look after the individual's needs, and possibly manage behavioural disturbance.

Prevention

This area has not been carefully investigated, but there are a number of natural experiments in the prevention of HIV associated dementia and related disorders. The first of them was the introduction of AZT, which was shown to be associated with a decrease in dementia. It is uncertain whether this is because it delays progression of the disease to AIDS or whether it arises from actual penetration of the drug and activity within the central nervous system (Portegies *et al.*, 1989). Another natural experiment was an epidemiological study in London; this revealed that when AZT use was decreased, there was an increase in the prevalence and incidence of HIV associated dementia.

The Future

When we consider the broad picture of HIV infection, any scientific advances that are made are likely to have a beneficial effect in HIV dementia. The virus itself might also change, making it more or less virulent, or possibly altering its tendency to infect the brain tissues and therefore the damage it causes. With more people who are HIV positive receiving treatment, the number of people who develop dementia may decrease, so fewer people may go on to suffer memory problems; or if they do, the problems may develop far more slowly. Even more new drug treatments may come from developments in understanding processes involved in the brain when dementia occurs. A number of specific advances have recently led to renewed optimism in the area of HIV dementia. Among them are the introduction of potent antiretroviral drugs and drug combinations and techniques to assay HIV-1 RNA in the blood; these assays have allowed more accurate means of assessing the severity of the HIV infection in different parts of the body.

The new drugs have raised the possibility of very long-term suppression, even eradication, of AIDS virus. They partly restore the CD4 count, decrease the incidence of opportunistic complications and prolong life. The cerebrospinal fluid (CSF) which surrounds the brain is sealed from the blood by membranes, which makes it difficult for many substances to enter the brain. This is usually protective, but it may cause problems when drugs are unable to enter. A number of existing drugs penetrate the cerebrospinal fluid in quantities that are insufficient to remove the virus completely. This allows the virus to continue to replicate and even to develop resistance to the drugs more rapidly. Thus the brain is very susceptible to the damaging presence of the virus. Assessment of the viral load of the CSF as well as existing measures of blood viral load, may, in future, assist clinicians to treat HIV optimally in respect of brain problems.

The development of drugs that can pass into the brain is important in this matter (Price and Staprans, 1997). Most recently there has been research from two centres which suggests that people with HIV who develop Kaposi's sarcoma may be protected from the development of any central nervous system disease, including the development of HIV-1 dementia. It is postulated that substances produced in the presence of Kaposi's sarcoma may block infection of microglial cells in the central nervous system, therefore having a neuroprotective effect (Baldeweg, Catalán and Gazzard, 1998; Liestrol *et al.*, 1998). These findings have implications for the understanding of why certain people develop HIV dementia whereas others do not, and they could lead to new ways of treating the problem.

References

AMERICAN ACADEMY of NEUROLOGY AIDS TASK FORCE (1991) 'Nomenclature and research case definitions for neurologic manifestations of HIV-1 infection', *Neurology*, **41**, pp. 778–85.

ANON (1990) 'World Health Organisation consultation on the neuropsychiatric aspects of HIV-1 infection, Geneva Jan 11–13, 1990', *AIDS*, **4**, pp. 935–36.

AYLWARD, E.H., HENDERER, J.D., MCARTHUR, J.C., BRETTSCHNEIDER, P.D., HARRIS, G.J., BARTA, P.E. *et al.* (1993) 'Reduced basal ganglia volume in

HIV-1-associated dementia: results from quantitative neuroimaging', *Neurology*, **43**, pp. 2099–2104.

BACELLAR, H., MUNOZ, A., MILLER, E. *et al.* (1994) 'Temporal trends in the incidence of HIV-1 related neurological diseases: multicentre AIDS cohort study', *Neurology*, **44**, pp. 1892–1900.

BALDEWEG, T., CATALÁN, J. and GAZZARD, B.G. (1998) 'Reduced risk of HIV dementia and opportunistic brain disease in AIDS associated with zidovudine use for up to 18 months', *Journal of Neurology*, **65**, pp. 34–41.

BELEC, L., MARTIN, P., VOHITO, M. and GRESENGUET, G. (1989) 'Low prevalence of neuropsychiatric clinical manifestations in Central African patients with AIDS', *Transactions of the Royal Society of Tropical Medicine and Hygiene*, **83**, pp. 844–46.

BELMAN, A.L., ULTMANN, M., HOROUPIAN, D., NOVICK, B.E., SPIRO, A.J., RUBINSTEIN, A. *et al.* (1985) 'Neurological complications in infants and children with acquired immune deficiency syndrome', *Annals of Neurology*, **18**, pp. 560–66.

BONI, J., EMMERICH, B.S., LEIB, S.L., WIESTLER, O.D., SCHUPBACH, J. and KLEIHUES, P. (1993) 'PCR identification of HIV-1 DNA sequences in brain tissue of patients with AIDS encephalopathy', *Neurology*, **43**, pp. 1813–17.

BREITBART, W., MAROTTA, R., PLATT, M.M., WEISMAN, H., DEREVENCO, M., GRAU, C., CORBERRA, K., LUND, S. and JACOBSEN, P. (1996) 'A double blind trial of haloperidol, chlorpromazine and lorazepam in the treatment of delirium in hospitalized AIDS patients', *American Journal of Psychiatry*, **153**, pp. 231–37.

BREW, B.J., BHALLA, R.B., FLEISHER, M., PAUL, M., KHAN, A., SCHWARTZ, M.K. *et al.* (1989) 'Cerebrospinal fluid β_2 microglobulin in patients infected with human immunodeficiency virus', *Neurology*, **39**, pp. 830–34.

BREW, B.J., BHALLA, R.B., PAUL, M., GALLARDO, H., McARTHUR, J.C., SCHWARTZ, M.K. *et al.* (1990) 'Cerebrospinal fluid neopterin in human immunodeficiecny virus type 1 infection', *Annals of Neurology*, **28**, pp. 556–60.

BUDKA, H., COSTANI, G., CRISTINA, S., LECHI, A., PARRAVICINI, C., TRABATTONI, R. *et al.* (1987) 'Brain pathology induced by infection with human immunodeficiency virus (HIV): a histological, immunocytochemical and electron microscopical study of 100 autopsy cases', *Acta Neuropathologica*, **75**, pp. 185–98.

BUDKA, H., WILEY, C.A., KLEIHUES, P., ARTIGAS, J., ASBURY, A.K., CHO, E.S. *et al.* (1991) 'HIV-associated disease of the nervous system: review of nomenclature and proposal for neuropathology-based terminology', *Brain Pathology*, **1**, pp. 143–52.

BURGESS, A.P. and THORNTON, S. (1995) 'Domains of the Charing Cross and Westminster Unit of Psychological Medicine Neuropsychological Battery', in Catalán, J., Burgess, A. and Klimes, I. (eds) *Psychological Medicine of HIV Infection*, Oxford: Oxford University Press.

BUTTERS, N., GRANT, I., HAXBY, J., JUDD, L.L., MARTIN, A., MCCLELLAND, J. *et al.* (1990) 'Assessment of AIDS related cognitive changes: recommendations of the NIMH workshop on neuropsychological assessment approaches', *Journal of Clinical and Experimental Neuropsychology*, **12**, pp. 963–78.

CANTACUZINO, M. (1993) *Till break of day*, London: Heinemann.

CATALÁN, J., BURGESS, A. and KLIMES, I. (1995) *Psychological Medicine of HIV Infection*, Oxford: Oxford University Press.

CHIESI, A., VELLA, S., DALLY, L.G., PEDERSON, C., DANNER, S., JOHNSON, A.M. *et al.* (1996) 'Epidemiology of AIDS dementia complex in Europe study group', *Journal of Acquired Immune Deficiency Syndrome and Human Retrovirology*, **11**, pp. 39–44.

CHOI, D.W. (1988) 'Calcium-mediated neurotoxicity: relationship to specific channel types and role in ischaemic damage', *Trends in Neuroscience*, **11**, pp. 465–69.

CVETKOVITCH, T.A., LAZAR, E., BLUMBERG, B.M., SAITO, Y., ESKIN, T.A., REICHMAN, R. *et al.* (1992) 'Human immunodeficiency virus type 1 infection of neural xenographs', *Proceedings of the National Academy of Science USA*, **11**, pp. 5162–66.

DAL PAN, G., GLASS, J. and MCARTHUR, J. (1994) 'Clinicopathological correlations of HIV-1 associated vacuolar myelopathy: an autopsy-cased case-controlled study', *Neurology*, **44**, pp. 2159–64.

DAL PAN, G.J., MCARTHUR, J.H., AYLWARD, E., SELNES, O.A., NANCE-SPROSON, T.E., KUMAR, A.J. *et al.* (1992) 'Patterns of cerebral atrophy in HIV-1-infected individuals: results of a quantitative MRI analysis', *Neurology*, **42**, pp. 2125–30.

DAVIS, L.E., HJELLE, B.J., MILLER, V.E., PALMER, D.L., LLEWELLYN, A.L., MERLIN, T.L. *et al.* (1992) 'Early viral brain invasion in iatrogenic human immunodeficiency virus infection', *Neurology*, **42**, pp. 1736–39.

DE GANS, J. and PORTEGIES, P. (1989) 'Neurological complications of infection with HIV-1', *Clinical Neurology and Neurosurgery*, **91**, pp. 199–219.

DERIX, M.M., DE GANS, J., STAM, J. and PORTEGIES, P. (1990) 'Mental changes in patients with AIDS', *Clinical Neurological Neurosurgery*, **92**, pp. 215–22.

DIAMOND, G.W., KAUFMAN, J., BELMAN, A.L., COHEN, L., COHEN, H.J. and RUBINSTEIN, A. (1987) 'Characterisation of cognitive functioning in a subgroup of children with congenital HIV infection', *Archives of Clinical Neuropsychiatry*, **2**, pp. 1–16.

DICKSON, D.W., LEE, S.C., HATCH, W., MATTIACE, L.A., BROSNAN, C.F. and LYMAN, W.D. (1994) 'Macrophages and microglia in HIV-related CNS neuropathology', *Research Publications of the Association for Research in Nervous and Mental Disease*, **72**, pp. 99–118.

DREYER, E.B., KAISER, P.K., OFFERMAN, J.T. and LIPTON, S.A. (1990) 'HIV-1 coat protein neurotoxicity prevented by calcium channel antagonists', *Science*, **248**, pp. 364–67.

EGAN, V., CRAWFORD, J.R., BRETTLE, R.P. and GOODWIN, G.M. (1990) 'The Edinburgh cohort of HIV positive drug users: current intellectual function is impaired, but not due to early AIDS dementia complex', *AIDS*, **4**, pp. 651–56.

EPSTEIN, L.G. and GENDELMAN, H.E. (1993) 'Human immunodeficiency virus type 1 infection of the nervous system: pathogenetic mechanisms', *Annals of Neurology*, **33**, pp. 429–36.

EPSTEIN, L.G., SHARER, L.R., OLESKE, J.M., CONNOR, E.M., GOUDSMIT, J., BAGDON, L. *et al.* (1986) 'Neurologic manifestations of HIV infection in children', *Paediatrics*, **78**, pp. 678–87.

ESIRI, M.M., SCARAVILLI, P.R., MILLARD, P.R. and HARCOURT-WEBSTER, J.N. (1990) 'Neuropathology of HIV infection in haemophiliacs: comparative necroscopy study', *British Medical Journal*, **299**, pp. 1312–15.

ESTERSON, A., HARRIS, H. and KESSINGER, J. (1992) 'The AIDS dementia unit', paper presented at the Eighth International Conference on AIDS, Amsterdam.

EVERALL, I. (1995) 'Neuropsychiatric aspects of HIV infection' *Journal of Neurology, Neurosurgery and Psychiatry*, **58**, pp. 399–402.

EVERALL, I., LUTHERT, P.J. and LANTOS, P.L. (1991) 'Neuronal loss in the frontal cortex in HIV infection', *Lancet*, **337**, pp. 1119–21.

EVERALL, I., LUTHERT, P.J. and LANTOS, P.L. (1993) 'Neuronal number and volume alterations in the neocortex of HIV infected individuals', *Journal of Neurology, Neurosurgery and Psychiatry*, **56**, pp. 481–86.

FERNANDEZ, F. and LEVY, J. (1990) 'Psychiatric diagnosis and pharmacotherapy of patients with HIV infection', *Review of Psychiatry*, **9**, pp. 614–30.

FLORENCE, M. (1994) 'Noah's Ark–Red Cross Foundation: a Swedish model', *AIDS Care*, **5**, pp. 467–70.

FOUDRAINE, N.A., HOETELMANS, R.M.W., LANGE, J.M.A., DE WOLF, F., VAN BENTHEM, B.H.B., MAAS, J.J., KEET, I.P.M. and PORTEGIES, P. (1998) 'Cerebrospinal-fluid HIV-1 RNA and drug concentrations after treatment with lamivudine plus zidovudine or stavudine', *Lancet*, **351**, pp. 1547–51.

GENIS, P., JETT, M., BERNTON, E.W., BOYLE, T., GELBARD, H.A., DZENKO, K. *et al.* (1992) 'Cytokines and arachidonic metabolites produced during human immunodeficiency virus (HIV) infected macrophage–astroglial interactions: implications for the neuropathogenesis of HIV disease', *Journal of Experimental Medicine*, **176**, pp. 1703–18.

GLASS, J.D., WESSELINGH, S.L., SELNES, O.A. and MCARTHUR, J.C. (1993) 'Clinical–neuropathological correlation in HIV associated dementia', *Neurology*, **43**, pp. 2230–37.

GOULSMITH, J., DE WOLF, F., PAUL, D.A., EPSTEIN, L.G., LANGE, J.M., KRONE, W.J. *et al.* (1996) 'Expression of human immunodeficiency virus antigen (HIV-Ag) in serum and cerebrospinal fluid during acute and chronic infection', *Lancet*, **2**, pp. 177–80.

GRANT, I., ATKINSON, H.J., HESSELINK, J.R., KENNEDY, C.J., RICHMAN, D.D., SPECTOR, S.A. *et al.* (1987) 'Evidence for early central nervous system involvement in the acquired immunodeficiency syndrome (AIDS) and other human immunodeficiency virus (HIV) infections. Studies with neuropsychologic testing and magnetic resonance imaging', *Annals of Internal Medicine*, **107**, pp. 828–36.

GRAY, F., LESCS, M., KEOHANE, C., PARAIRE, F., MARC, B., DURIGON, M. *et al.* (1992) 'Early brain changes in HIV infection: neuropathological study of 11 HIV seropositive, non-AIDS cases', *Journal of Neuropathology and Experimental Neurology*, **51**, pp. 177–85.

GREEN, J. and KOCSIS, A. (1988) 'Counselling patients with AIDS related encephalopathy', *Journal of the Royal College of Physicians of London*, **22**, pp. 166–68.

GRIMALDI, L.M., MARTINO, G.V., FRANCIOTTA, D.M., BRUSTIA, R., CASTAGNA, A., PRISTERA, R. *et al.* (1991) 'Elevated alpha-tumor necrosis factor levels in spinal fluid from HIV-1 infected patients with central nervous system involvement', *Annals of Neurology*, **29**, pp. 21–25.

HARDEN, C.L., DARAS, M., TUCHMAN, A.J. and KOPPEL, B.S. (1993) Low amplitude EEGs in demented AIDS patients', *Electroencephalography and Clinical Neurophysiology*, **87**, pp. 54–55.

HEYES, M.P., RUBINOW, D., LANE, C. and MARKEY, S.P. (1989) 'Cerebrospinal fluid quinolinic acid concentrations are increased in acquired immune deficiency syndrome', *Annals of Neurology*, **26**, pp. 275–77.

HEYES, M.P., MEFFORD, I.N., QUEARRY, B.J., DEDHIA, M. and LACKNER, A. (1990) 'Increased ratio of quinolinic acid to kynurenic acid in cerebrospinal fluid of D retrovirus-infected rhesus macaques: relationship to clinical and viral status', *Annals of Neurology*, **27**, pp. 666–75.

HEYES, M.P., BREW, B.J., MARTIN, A., PRICE, R.W., SALAZAR, A.M., SIDTIS, J.J. *et al.* (1991) 'Quinolinic acid in cerebrospinal fluid and serum in HIV-1 infection: relationship to clinical and neurological status', *Annals of Neurology*, **29**, pp. 202–9.

HO, D.D., ROTA, T.R., SCHOOLEY, R.T., KAPLAN, J.C., ALLAN, J.D., GROOPMANAA, J.E. *et al.* (1985) 'Isolation of HTLV-III from cerebrospinal fluid and neural tissues of patients with neurologic syndromes related to acquired immune deficiency syndrome', *New England Journal of Medicine*, **313**, pp. 1493–97.

HOWLETT, W.P., NKYA, V.M., NMUMI, K.A. and MISSALELE, W.R. (1989) 'Neurologic disorders in AIDS and HIV disease in the northern zone of Tanzania', *AIDS*, **3**, pp. 289–96.

HRISO, E., KUHN, T., MASDEU, J. and GRUNDMAN, M. (1991) 'Extrapyramidal symptoms due to dopamine blocking agents in patients with AIDS encephalopathy', *American Journal of Psychiatry*, **148**, pp. 1558–61.

KETZLER, S., WEISS, S., HAUG, H. and BUDKA, H. (1990) 'Loss of neurones in the frontal cortex in AIDS brains', *Acta Neuropathology (Berlin)*, **80**, pp. 92–94.

Kocsis, A. (1989) 'Counselling those with AIDS dementia', in Green, J. and McCreaner, A. (eds) *Counselling in HIV infection and AIDS*, Oxford: Blackwell Scientific.

Lantos, P.L., McLaughlin, J.E., Scholtz, C.L., Berry, C.L. and Tighe, J.R. (1989) 'Neuropathology of the brain in HIV infection', *Lancet*, **i**, pp. 309–11.

Lenhardt, T.M., Super, M.A. and Wiley, C.A. (1988) 'Neuropathological changes in an asymptomatic HIV seropositive man', *Annals of Neurology*, **23**, pp. 209–10.

Liestoel, K., Golpen, A.K., Dunlop, O., Bruun, J. and Moehlen, J. (1998) 'Kaposi's sarcoma and protection from HIV dementia', *Science*, **280**, p. 361.

Lipton, S.A., Sucher, N.J., Kaiser, P.K. and Dreyer, E.B. (1991) 'Synergistic effects of the HIV coat protein and NMDA receptor-mediated neurotoxicity, *Neuron*, **7**, pp. 111–18.

Lyketsos, C.G., Hanson, A., Fishman, M., Rosenblatt, A., McHugh, P. and Treisman, D. (1993) 'Manic syndrome early and late in the course of HIV', *American Journal of Psychiatry*, **150**, pp. 326–27.

Lyketsos, C.G., Schwartz, J., Fishman, M. and Treisman, D. (1997) 'AIDS mania', *Journal of Neuropsychiatry*, **9**, 2, 277–79.

McArthur, J.C. (1987) 'Neurologic manifestations of AIDS', *Medicine*, **66**, pp. 407–37.

McArthur, J.C., Cohen, B.A., Farzedegan, H., Cornblath, D.R., Selnes, D.A., Ostrow, D. *et al* (1988) 'Cerebrospinal fluid abnormalities in homosexual men with and without neuropsychiatric findings', *Annals of Neurology*, **23**, pp. s34–37.

McArthur, J.C., Nance-Sprosen, T.E., Griffin, D.E., Hoover, D., Selnes, O.A., Miller, E.N. *et al.* (1992) 'The diagnostic utility of elevation in cerebrospinal fluid β_2 microglobulin in HIV-1 dementia: multicenter AIDS cohort study', *Neurology*, **42**, pp. 1707–12.

McArthur, J.C., Hoover, D.R., Bacellar, H., Miller, E.N., Cohen, B.A. and Becker, J.T. (1993) 'Dementia in AIDS patients: incidence and risk factors', *Neurology*, **43**, pp. 2245–52.

Maj, M., Janssen, R. and Satz, P. (1991) 'The WHO cross-cultural study on neuropsychiatric aspects of HIV-1 infection: preparation and pilot phase', *British Journal of Psychiatry*, **159**, pp. 351–56.

Maj, M., Janssen, R., Starace, F., Zaudig, M., Satz, P. and Sughondhabirom, B. (1994a) 'WHO neuropsychiatric AIDS study – cross-sectional phase', *Archives of General Psychiatry*, **51**, pp. 39–49.

Maj, M., Satz, P., Janssen, R., Zaudig, M., Starace, F. and D'Elia, L. (1994b) 'WHO neuropsychiatric AIDS study – cross-sectional phase: neuropsychological and neurological findings', *Archives of General Psychiatry*, **51**, pp. 51–61.

Masliah, E., Achim, C.L., Ge, N., DeTeresa, R., Terry, R.D. and Wiley,

C.A. (1992) 'Spectrum of human immunodeficiency virus – associated neocortical damage', *Annals of Neurology*, **32**, pp. 321–29.

MAYEUX, R., STERN, Y., TANG, M., TODAK, G., MARDER, K. and SANO, M. (1993) 'Mortality risk in gay men with HIV infection and cognitive impairment', *Neurology*, **43**, pp. 176–82.

MEADOWS, J. and CATALÁN, J. (1994) 'The needs of carers of patients with chronic brain disorders in HIV disease in the Thames regions, London', paper presented at AIDS' Impact II, Brighton.

MEILLET, D., BELEC, L., CELTON, N. *et al.* (1993) 'Intrathecal synthesis of β_2-microglobulin and lysozyme: differential markers of nervous system involvement in patients infected with human immunodeficiency virus type 1', *European Journal of Clinical Chemistry and Clinical Biochemistry*, **31**, 10, 609–15.

MICHAELS, J., SHARER, L.R. and EPSTEIN, L.G. (1988) 'Human immunodeficiency virus type one (HIV-1) infection of the nervous system: a review', *Immunodeficiency Review*, **1**, pp. 71–104.

NAVIA, B. (1990) 'The AIDS dementia complex', in Cummings, J.L. (ed.) *Subcortical Dementia*, New York: Oxford University Press, pp. 181–88.

NAVIA, B.A., JORDAN, B.D. and PRICE, R.W. (1986) 'The AIDS dementia complex, I: clinical features', *Annals of Neurology*, **19**, pp. 517–24.

NAVIA, B.A., CHO, E.S., PETITO, C.K. and PRICE, R.W. (1986) 'The AIDS dementia complex, II: neuropathology', *Annals of Neurology*, **19**, pp. 525–35.

O'BRIEN, W. (1994) 'Genetic and biologic basis of HIV-1 neurotropism', in Price, R. and Perry, S. (eds) *HIV, AIDS and the Brain*, New York: Raven, pp. 47–70.

OLSEN, W.L., LONGO, F.M., MILLS, C.M. and NORMAN, D. (1988) 'White matter disease in AIDS: findings at MR imaging', *Radiology*, **169**, pp. 445–48.

OSTROW, D., GRANT, I. and ATKINSON, J.H. (1988) 'Assessment and management of the AIDS patient with neuropsychiatric disturbance', *Journal of Clinical Psychiatry*, **49**, pp. 14–22.

OSTROW, D., HARRIS, H. and MILL, K. (1992) 'Assessing a new model of inpatient subacute care for HIV related dementia', paper presented at the Eighth International Conference on AIDS, Amsterdam.

PANG, S., KOYANAGI, Y., MILES, S., WILEY, C., VINTERS, H.V. and CHEN, I.S. (1990) 'High levels of unintegrated HIV-1 DNA in brain tissue of AIDS dementia patients', *Nature*, **343**, pp. 85–89.

PARISI, A., STROSSELLI, M. and DI PERRI, G. (1988) 'EEE in the early diagnosis of HIV-related subacute encephalitis: analysis of 185 patients', *Clinical Electroencephalography*, **20**, pp. 1–5.

PELUSO, R., HAASE, A., STOWRING, L., EDWARDS, M. and VENTURA, P. (1985) 'A Trojan Horse mechanism for the spread of venisa virus in monocytes', *Virology*, **147**, pp. 231–36.

PERRIENS, J.H., MUSSA, M., LUABEYA, M.K., KAYEMBE, K., KAPITA, B., BROWN,

C. *et al.* (1992) 'Neurologic complications of HIV-1 seropositive internal medicine patients in Kinshasa, Zaire', *Journal of Acquired Immune Deficiency Syndromes*, **5**, pp. 333–40.

PERT, C.B., SMITH, C.C., RUFF, M.R. and HILL, J.M. (1988) 'AIDS and its dementia as a neuropeptide disorder: role of VIP receptor blockade by human immunodeficiency virus envelope', *Annals of Neurology*, **23**, pp. s71–73.

PETITO, C.K., CHO, E.S., LEMANN, W., NAVIA, B.A. and PRICE, R.W. (1986) 'Neuropathology of AIDS: an autopsy review', *Journal of Neuropathology and Experimental Neurology*, **45**, pp. 643–46.

PETTITO, C.K. and CASH, K.S. (1992) 'Blood–brain barrier abnormalities in the acquired immunodeficiency syndrome: immunohistochemical localization of serum proteins in postmortem brain', *Annals of Neurology*, **32**, pp. 658–66.

PORTEGIES, P., DE GANS, J., LANGE, J.M., DERIX, M., SPEELMAN, H. and BAKKER, M. (1989) 'Declining incidence of ADC after introduction of AZT treatment', *British Medical Journal*, **299**, pp. 819–21.

PORTEGIES, P., ENTING, R.H., DE GANS, J., ALGRA, P.R., DERIX, M.M., LANGE, J.M. *et al.* (1993) 'Presentation and course of AIDS dementia complex: 10 years of follow-up in Amsterdam, the Netherlands', *AIDS*, **7**, pp. 669–75.

POST, M.J., TATE, L.G., QUENCER, R.M., HENSLEY, G.T., BERGER, J.R., SHEREMATA, W.A. *et al.* (1988) 'CT, MR and pathology in HIV encephalitis and meningitis', *American Journal of Roentgenology*, **151**, pp. 373–80.

POWER, C., KONG, P.A., CRAWFORD, T.O., WESSELINGH, S., GLASS, J.D., MCARTHUR, J.C. *et al.* (1993) 'Cerebral white matter changes in acquired immunodeficency syndrome dementia: alteration of the blood–brain barrier', *Annals of Neurology*, **34**, pp. 339–50.

PRICE, R.W. (1995) 'Managment of AIDS dementia complex and HIV-1 infection of the nervous system', *AIDS*, **9**, suppl. A, pp. 221–36.

PRICE, R.W. (1996) 'Neurological complications of HIV infection', *Lancet*, **348**, pp. 445–52.

PRICE, R.W. and BREW, B.J. (1988) 'AIDS commentary: the AIDS dementia complex', *Journal of Infectious Diseases*, **158**, pp. 1079–83.

PRICE, R.W. and STAPRANS, S. (1997) 'Measuring the "viral load" in cerebrospinal fluid in human immunodeficiency virus infection: window into brain infection?', *Annals of Neurology*, **42**, 5, pp. 675–78.

SACKTOR, N.C., BACELLAR, H., HOOVER, D.R., NANCE-SPROSON, T.E., SELNES, O.A., MILLER, E.N. *et al.* (1996) 'Psychomotor slowing in HIV infection: a predictor of dementia, AIDS and death', *Journal of Neurovirology*, **2**, pp. 404–10.

SCURLOCK, H., SINGH, A. and CATALÁN, J. (1995) 'Atypical antipsychotic drugs in the treatment of manic syndromes in HIV-1 infection', *Journal of Psychopharmacology*, **9**, 2, pp. 151–54.

SEILHEAN, D., DUYCKAERTS, C., VAZEUX, R., BOLGERT, F., BRUNET, P.,

KATLAMA, C. *et al.* (1993) 'HIV-1-associated cognitive/motor complex: absence of neuronal loss in the cerebral neocortex', *Neurology*, **43**, pp. 1492–99.

SELNES, O.A., McARTHUR, J.C., McARTHUR, J.H. and SAAH, A. (1991) 'Incidence of HIV dementia in the MACS: patterns of cognitive decline', paper presented at the International Conference on the Neuroscience of HIV Infection, Padua.

SELNES, O.A., McARTHUR, J.C., ROYAL, W. III, UPDIKE, M.L., NANCE-SPOROSON, T., CONCHA, M. *et al.* (1992) 'HIV-1 infection and intravenous drug use: longitudinal neuropsychological evaluation of asymptommatic subjects', *Neurology*, **42**, pp. 1924–30.

SHAW, G.M., HARPER, M.E., HAHN, B.H., EPSTEIN, L.G., GAJDUSEK, D.C., PRICE, R.W. *et al.* (1985) 'HTLV-III infections in brains of children and adults with AIDS encephalopathy', *Science*, **227**, pp. 177–82.

SIDTIS, J.J., AMITAI, H., ORNITZ, D. and PRICE, R.W. (1988) 'Neuropsychological and neurological characterisation of the AIDS dementia complex', *Journal of Clinical Experimental Neuropsychology*, **10**, p. 76.

SIMPSON, D.M. and TAGLIATI, M. (1994) 'Neurologic manifestations of HIV infection', *Annals of Internal Medicine*, **121**, pp. 769–85.

SIMS, R. and MOSS, V. (1991) *Terminal Care for People with AIDS*, London: Edward Arnold.

SINGH, A. and CATALÁN, J. (1994) 'Risperidone in HIV related manic psychosis', *Lancet*, **344**, pp. 1029–30.

SNIDER, W.D., SIMPSON, D.M., NIELSON, S., GOLD, J.W.M., METROKA, C.E. and POSNER, J.B. (1983) 'Neurological complications of AIDS: analysis of 50 patients', *Annals of Neurology*, **14**, pp. 403–18.

TROSS, S., PRICE, R.W., NAVIA, B.A., THALER, H.T., GOLD, J., HIRSCH, D.A. *et al.* (1988) 'Neuropsychological characterisation of the AIDS dementia complex: a preliminary report', *AIDS*, **2**, pp. 81–88.

VAN GORP, W.G., MILLER, E.N., MARCHOTTE, T.D., DIXON, W., PAZ, D., SELNES, O. *et al.* (1994) 'The relationship between age cognitive impairment in HIV-1 infections: findings from the multicentre AIDS cohort study and a clinical cohort', *Neurology*, **44**, pp. 929–35.

WESSELINGH, S.L., POWER, C., GLASS, J.D., TYOR, W.R., McARTHUR, J.C., FARBER, J.M. *et al.* (1993) 'Intracerebral cytokine messenger RNA expression in acquired immunodeficiency syndrome dementia', *Annals of Neurology*, **33**, 576–82.

WILEY, C.A., MASLIAH, F. and MOREY, M. (1991) 'Neocortical damage during HIV infection', *Annals of Neurology*, **29**, pp. 651–57.

WORLD HEALTH ORGANIZATION (1990) *Report of the Second Consultation on the Neuropsychiatric Aspects of HIV-1 Infection*, Geneva: WHO.

Chapter 6

Suicidal Behaviour and HIV Infection

Carole Mitchell

People infected with HIV are likely to experience psychological as well as physical problems during the course of their illness. For some, this becomes too much to bear and it can result in suicide. There are others who consider harming themselves but who may never act on these thoughts. The effect of this on their quality of life, however, can be considerable. It is therefore important that we improve our understanding of suicidal behaviour so that we can detect and help those who may be at risk. This chapter identifies characteristics of patients at risk of suicide using what we have learned from the recent research in this area and also describes the steps in assessing and offering support to reduce the likelihood of suicide.

Introduction

The association between HIV infection and suicide has continued to attract attention from researchers over the last decade. Given the complexity of the issues involved in suicidal behaviour, disagreement has arisen on the conclusions of some of these studies. The heterogeneity of the studies has made it difficult to draw generalized conclusions because of the differences in the populations studied.

Methodological problems have made it difficult to establish whether HIV infection in itself results in suicidality as an 'inducer' or 'catalyst' (Marzuk and Perry, 1993) or whether other variables come into play. Some studies have failed to match controls by sexual orientation or drug use, which in themselves are known to increase suicidality. Therefore results from these studies may give a falsely high level of suicidal behaviour in people with HIV. On the other hand, the hidden nature of suicide, inaccurate AIDS statistics and misclassified deaths may mean that we are only seeing the tip of the iceberg.

There have been some attempts to identify which psychosocial factors are more likely to predispose to suicidal behaviour. Given the many stresses on people with HIV, it is too simplistic to assume that infection with HIV is the sole cause of their suicidality. Certainly, HIV infection can be a source of multiple stressors, particularly those known to be associated with suicidal risk. HIV infection brings the awareness of an uncertain future with an arguably incurable illness. Those infected find that their lives are affected forever and in many areas. They are more likely to suffer bereavements of close friends and partners and suffer losses: financial, work and health. Their relationships can be affected and some find themselves isolated and stigmatized. HIV-infected people often have other risk factors such as substance misuse, previous psychiatric problems and poor social support predating infection with the virus (Perry, Jacobsberg and Fishman, 1990). Although the epidemic is spreading to affect all facets of society, the majority of those infected in developed countries are still predominantly gay men and intravenous drug misusers. There is some evidence to suggest that these groups already have a higher rate of suicidal behaviour than the general population (Schneider *et al.*, 1991; Klee, 1995).

It is important not to compare studies of suicidal ideators with suicidal completers as they may belong to distinct but overlapping populations (Linehan, 1986). Not all people involved in acts of self-harm wish to die. Very often the motivation is to express emotional distress. Also, not everyone completing suicide had that intent. Therefore, in the research review, three groups will be discussed and illustrated by case studies: suicidal ideation, attempted suicide and completed suicide.

Suicidal Ideation

Prevalence

Most studies of suicidal ideation focus on people with AIDS. However, in one study of asymptomatic individuals presenting for an HIV test, a high level of suicidal ideation was found in the lead-up to testing in almost one-third of patients (Perry, Jacobsberg and Fishman, 1990). This was equally high in the HIV positive and the HIV negative groups. Only those later diagnosed as HIV positive maintained this level of suicidality (27 per cent at 1 week and 16 per cent at 2 months) whereas the suicidal ideas in the HIV negative group decreased rapidly to 17 per cent at 1 week follow-up. The authors therefore argued that the prevalence of suicidal ideation is raised in HIV-infected individuals, but added that suicidal thoughts did not increase following notification of a positive result.

Rabkin *et al.* (1993) reported a low rate of mood disorders and hopelessness in long-term AIDS survivors, with many reporting a high level of well-being. While 57 per cent of this group admitted to having had thoughts of ending their lives; these seemed to occur in the context of acute illness and only 2 out of the 53 men had made an attempt since knowing of their AIDS diagnosis. Others disagree that the level of suicidal thinking is high. O'Dowd *et al.* (1989) did not find an increase in suicidal ideation or attempts in those with HIV-related disease. In later studies by this same group, AIDS patients were found to have less suicidal ideation than those with asymptomatic HIV infection, and it was suggested that one of the reasons may be the increased organicity seen in AIDS patients.

It is difficult to draw any firm conclusions from these differing results. This is perhaps an example of the complex nature of suicide and how we must be careful not to apply the same rules to individuals in different settings or at different stages of infection.

Precipitants

The timing of maximal suicidal ideation appears to vary with the course of the disease (Sherr, 1995). These ideas seem to occur at specific stages. They tend to occur soon after the initial HIV diagnosis and again when the diagnosis of AIDS is made. Likewise, the first episode of illness can have a profound psychological impact.

Certain triggers precipitate suicidal thinking in HIV-infected people. These include bereavement and episodes of mental disorder, such as depression, anxiety, psychosis and delirium. The most common link between those considering suicide is that they are more likely to have a past psychiatric history and have made previous suicide attempts (Rabkin *et al.*, 1993). Others have noted the effect of cumulative stressors and poor social support (Rabkin *et al.*, 1990). In other populations hopelessness appears to be a key feature in those contemplating suicide (Beck, Kovacs and Weissman, 1975). It is also known to be high in gay men and men with haemophilia and HIV, and therefore may act as an indicator of suicidality (Catalán *et al.*, 1992). However, hopelessness has been shown elsewhere to become less prominent as health deteriorates (Rabkin *et al.*, 1993). There are a variety of possible explanations for this. It may be due to denial or that a diagnosis of AIDS brings a new sense of the value of life, or perhaps even that CNS (central nervous system) changes are involved.

Highlighting the importance of looking at not just HIV diagnosis itself, but the many effects this can have on peoples lives, suicidal ideation in partners of men with AIDS has been found to relate more to bereavement than to their own HIV status (Rosengard and Folkman, 1997). Over half the primary caregivers of gay and bisexual men with AIDS in this study admitted to suicidal ideation. They were more likely to have suicidal thoughts if they experienced a feeling of being burdened as a caregiver, perceived a lack of social support or used escape-avoidance coping strategies. In Case 6.1 suicidal ideation was a clear indicator of a depressive illness, rather than a normal understandable reaction to John's situation. Case 6.1 also illustrates the beneficial effects of psychological and psychopharmacological interventions.

Case 6.1

John is a 39-year-old gay man who was given an AIDS diagnosis at the same time as his HIV diagnosis in 1986. His CD4 count at the time of referral (1997) to psychiatric services was 57 and his viral load was 385. He had already had three AIDS-defining illnesses by this time (PCP, MAI and encephalopathy) and he had just been started on treatment with AZT, lamivudine (3TC) and indinavir.

He had initially been referred by his HIV physician, who thought he may benefit from seeing the liaison psychiatric nurse. He had also been recently prescribed diazepam by his GP. Following an initial assessment, the nurse requested that a psychiatrist see the patient as she believed him to be depressed.

At the first appointment with the psychiatrist, John initially denied suicidal ideation, but as he discussed his past history, he soon became tearful and admitted that he often considered killing himself as a means of escaping his problems.

He had a history of depression one year previously, following the death of his partner by AIDS. He had been treated with anti-depressants by his GP but unfortunately, just as he was beginning to show a response, he developed encephalopathy and was admitted to hospital, where the antidepressant was stopped. His depressive symptoms lingered on and his suicidal ideation increased around the anniversary of his partner's death.

Initially he was very ambivalent about seeing a psychiatrist, stating that it made him more depressed as he felt he had 'hit rock bottom'. However, he continued to attend and was prescribed the antidepressant sertraline; he soon made a full recovery from his depression and suicidal ideation.

Attempted Suicide

Prevalence

Suicide attempts or deliberate self-harm (DSH) are commoner than completed suicide, but research in this area of HIV is more scarce. Also it is difficult to compare the results of these studies as they often use different stages of illness and study design. Depending on the population studied, different results have been found. For instance, neither attempted nor completed suicides were found among females in the United States Air Force (USAF) from 1987 to 1991 (Brown and Rundell, 1993). These results were considered to be related to the lower prevalence of psychiatric disorders among females, linked to the absence of conflicts about sexual orientation. Also, no suicide attempts were reported in a group of 37 HIV positive men with haemophilia (Catalán *et al.*, 1992). Therefore it is important to note the risk category to which people belong rather than apply generalizations to different groups.

Associated Risks

Many researchers agree that the risk of DSH in people with HIV infection is higher in individuals with a history of previous DSH, in those with a past psychiatric history, and in those with psychiatric disorders (Gala *et al.*, 1992).

Several examples exist to support this (Table 6.1). In a large study of 438 HIV positive and HIV negative patients attending an outpatient clinic, the number of previous attempts was greater in the seropositive group (Gala *et al.*, 1993). According to James, Rubin and Willis (1991), attempted suicide in pregnant women appears to be commoner in those who are drug dependent (21.1 per cent) compared to those who are not (2.8 per cent). Some patients directly blamed receiving the diagnosis of HIV as the reason for these previous attempts. In a 1995 study, only 6 of the 22 index cases stated that their previous DSH was related to HIV infection, and in the majority of cases the attempt was made before the diagnosis of HIV was known (Catalán *et al.*, 1995b).

Sherr (1995) demonstrated that while a high number of psychology clinic attendees had made an attempt since HIV diagnosis, a similar number had

Table 6.1 *Attempted suicide*

Study	Sample	Prenotification attempts	Post-notification attempts	Comments
Gala *et al.* (1992)	279 HIV+ asymptomatic	41 (15%)		more attempts in seropositive drug users
	159 HIV−	13 (8%)		
Catalan *et al.* (1995)	22 HIV+	10 (45%)		6 (23%) attributed the attempt to HIV
	44 HIV−	17 (37%)		
Sherr (1995)	41 HIV+	18 (43.9%)	17 (41.5%)	14.6% both pre- and post-notification
O'Dowd, Biderman and McKegney (1993)	183 HIV+	66 (36%)	10 (5.5%)	13.1% attempted at time of notification
Rabkin *et al.* (1993)	53 HIV+ (AIDS)	(23% attempted before AIDS diagnosis)[a]		

[a] Timing of attempt not specified.

attempted prior to diagnosis, suggesting that these patients are already vulnerable to suicidal behaviour. The incidence of attempts in O'Dowd's sample of outpatients with AIDS was 41.5 per cent (O'Dowd, Biderman and McKegney, 1993). The minority had made the attempt soon after HIV diagnosis and fewer still (6.6 per cent) actually attributed the attempt to this. This is an important point as we would have to reconsider the value of testing at all if it appeared that it was resulting in increased suicide attempts.

Past history of psychiatric problems also seems to predict attempts at self-harm. Gala *et al.* (1992) found the risk of DSH to be seven times greater in those with previous psychiatric problems. In particular, a history of depression appears to predispose people to risk of suicide attempts (Catalán *et al.*, 1995). Concerns about their physical health were also prominent among the HIV positive cases in Catalán's study. Psychiatric follow-up was offered more often to HIV subjects than controls. However, alcohol misuse was more often diagnosed in their seronegative group.

In Rundell's 1992 study of HIV positive attempters in the USAF, there was a different result (Rundell *et al.*, 1992) The attempters had more alcohol misuse, adjustment disorders and personality disorders. The diagnosis of a current major depression was minimal, whereas a history of major depression was significantly more frequent among attempters. In Spain a relatively low rate of suicidality was found in HIV positive patients referred to a liaison psychiatrist. Out of the 442 cases, 17 were reported to have made a suicide attempt, and again they noted that past psychiatric history and previous suicide attempts predicted a higher risk of suicidality (Carvajal *et al.*, 1995).

The motivation behind DSH is known to be different from the motivation in completed suicide. Often there is no intent to die but rather to escape an intolerable situation. Triggers of self-harm are often but not always HIV and AIDS related issues. Besides the link with past suicide attempt and current expressed suicidal ideation, other reasons given include bereavement, relationship problems, inability to cope with HIV/AIDS, waiting for the HIV result and trauma at the time of HIV testing (Sherr, 1995).

Timing

The timing of attempts may be linked to particular events related to HIV disease. Some have suggested a bimodal distribution of suicide attempts, dependent on the stage of infection. Sherr's study endorsed this idea, indicating peaks at or around diagnosis and a second peak at the time of AIDS illnesses. This may suggest that we need to address these issues and offer the appropriate interventions. In a selected sample of military airforce subjects, 47 per cent of attempts were committed within 3 months of diagnosis and 66.7 per cent within 1 year (Rundell *et al.*, 1992). Carvajal also noticed that the timing of attempts at self-harm centred around the onset of AIDS, recurrent illness and starting new HIV treatments (Carvajal *et al.*, 1995).

Methods Used in the Act of Self-Harm

Attempted suicide by violent methods such as gunshot or hanging had been shown elsewhere to be related to greater psychiatric morbidity and serious physical illness (Kontaxis *et al.*, 1988). Most of the studies in HIV have shown otherwise. The minority of people used the methods of drowning, hanging and cutting wrists in Sherr's 1995 study: 82 per cent attempted self-harm by taking an overdose. Catalán found a similar result: 81 per cent used overdose as the form of DSH and there was no difference in the control group (Catalán *et al.*, 1995). Case 6.2 illustrates that attempted suicide in those with HIV infection often occurs in the context of extreme stress which can be directly related to HIV itself; it also shows that frequently there are many other factors involved, including an underlying vulnerability to depression and suicidal behaviour.

Case 6.2

Gillian was a 36-year-old woman who was presented to psychiatric services when she was 30 weeks pregnant in 1993. She had been referred by her HIV physician for help with anxiety and insomnia. At that time she was known to be HIV positive with a CD4 count of 320 but had had no AIDS-defining illnesses.

The history given to the psychologist at assessment was that she had recently returned to the UK after a 10-year period living abroad. She had ended a three-year relationship with the father of her un-born child and now had no contact with him. The anxiety and insomnia had been worsening over the previous few months in anticipation of the impending birth, about which she was extremely ambivalent.

She had been diagnosed with HIV infection in 1987 and reported taking an overdose at that time in an attempt at suicide. She had made three previous similar attempts earlier in her life at times of crisis but denied any suicidal intention at the time of assessment. She also gave a history of previous bouts of depression during her life, for which she had sought counselling. She was estranged from her family and received little support from friends.

The psychologist embarked on a course of relaxation sessions with her and liaised with her social worker, who was helping her with housing and the possibility of providing foster care for her child. However, following the birth of her son Jack, Gillian decided to look after him at home herself and for a short period was happy. Unfortunately, quite soon after his birth, Jack became ill and was diagnosed with CMV infection. He was admitted to hospital and Gillian became increasingly despondent.

She was seen by a psychiatrist, who prescribed the antidepressant fluoxetine, and she continued to see the psychologist and her social worker for support. After about a month, her mood had improved but both her and her son's physical state began to deteriorate. Gillian developed oral candidiasis and Jack was again admitted for investigation of an enlarged liver. They both had a short stay in a respite care facility before returning home.

By September of 1994 it was becoming clear that Jack's prognosis was poor and Gillian talked about preparing for his death. Jack finally died in January of 1995. The months following this were extremely difficult for Gillian, and although she continued to see her psychologist, she denied any suicidal intention. However, one night, after drinking a bottle of wine and brandy, she took an overdose of ibuprofen and temazepam. She awoke the following day in her son's bedroom with little recollection of events.

She called for help and was admitted to the HIV inpatient unit. After a further period of respite care and ongoing support from both psychiatry and psychology, she returned home feeling calmer and seemed to be coming to terms more with Jack's death. Six months later she was given a diagnosis of AIDS, having developed oesophageal candidiasis, MAI and PCP. Her CD4 count had dropped to 4.

She continued the bereavement work with the psychologist and joined a bereavement group. She reported sleeping better and was dealing with her son's death better. By April of 1996 she had been diagnosed with cerebral lymphoma and she was resigned to an imminent death. She requested to be allowed to die at home and was provided with a 24-hour carer. Gillian died at home a month later.

Completed Suicide

It is difficult to identify suicidal deaths in any population given the secretive nature of the act. In completed suicides the cause of death is often misclassified and evidence as to the intent of the deceased unknown.

Prevalence

A number of researchers looking at completed suicides have argued over whether there is in fact an increase in suicidal deaths in individuals with HIV infection. Most studies have focused on those with AIDS, so very little data exists on asymptomatic HIV-infected subjects. Studies have also identified these cases retrospectively by death certificates or postmortem findings, which may not always be reliable indicators of suicidal intent or HIV status.

The association between a diagnosis of AIDS and the risk of suicide was initially reported to be increased by Marzuk *et al.* (1988). They identified 668 deaths by suicide in New York City in 1985. Twelve of these were known to have had AIDS: all male, aged 20–59 years, who died within 6 to 9 months of receiving an AIDS diagnosis. When compared to men of the same age and race, they were found to have a suicide risk that was 36 times greater. Marzuk believed that this underestimated the true figure (Table 6.2). Subsequent work by Kizer in California and Plott in Texas showed a similar increase – relative risk 17 times and 16 times greater, respectively. (Kizer *et al.*, 1988; Plott, Benton and Winslade, 1989). Cote, Biggar and Dannenberg (1992) found that the relative risk for suicide decreased over the three years of their study. In 1987 the risk was 10.5 times greater, falling to 6 times in 1989. They postulated that this may have been a sign of the optimism in the newer antivirals and prophylactic agents introduced at that time. Overall they found the relative risk (RR) to be 7.4 times that of the general population. However, they conceded that they should have compared these subjects to individuals within the same risk group. There have also been case reports published describing deaths from suicide in people known to be HIV positive but which do not give any accurate information on suicide risk compared to the general population (Pugh, O'Donnell and Catalán, 1993).

Some studies compare the AIDS-related suicides with the general population, failing to take into account the other risk factors for suicide pertaining to certain risk groups. The relative risk of suicide for homosexuals is thought to be higher than the general population (Schneider *et al.*, 1991). The increased mortality rate of drug users may also be due to suicidal deaths, although it has been difficult to accurately demonstrate suicidal intent in those who have overdosed (Klee, 1995). Starace (1995) argued that, unless this is taken into account, it may lead to an overestimation of suicide risk among AIDS patients.

In some centres, a low number of suicides have been reported. A prospective study by Dannenberg *et al.* (1996) followed 4,147 HIV positive military service applicants and 12,437 HIV negative applicants who had been discharged for other medical conditions from 1985 to 1993. They saw no signifi-

Table 6.2 *Completed suicide: studies showing increased risk*

Study	Centre	Cases of AIDS suicides	Adjusted RR[a]	General RR[b]
Marzuk *et al.* (1988)	New York	12	36×	66×
Kizer *et al.* (1988)	California	13	17×	21×
Plott, Benton and Winslade (1989)	Texas	13		16×
Cote, Biggar and Dannenberg (1992)	United States	165		7.4×[c]
Marzuk *et al.* (1997)	New York	133	2×	

[a] Relative risk adjusted for age and sex.
[b] Relative risk for the general population.
[c] Over 3 years.

cant difference in risk of death by suicide in this large sample. In 1995 Pueschel and Heineman published their work on HIV-related suicides in Hamburg. They reported that of the 93 HIV positive deaths from 1989 to 1994, 17 were by suicide. They found no increase in intravenous drug users compared to non-users. They concluded that a rate of 3 suicides per year was not high. Similarly, when studying 176 drug addict deaths in London from 1987 to 1992, Paterson, Vanezis and Claydon (1996) found no increase in the incidence of suicide in addicts who knew of their HIV positive status. A low incidence of suicide has also been found in people with haemophilia who are HIV infected. Jones (1995) suggested that the comprehensive care offered to this group may help to alleviate the factors contributing to suicide risk.

Methods Used in Completed Suicide

People take their lives in different ways. In early reports it seemed that jumping was the preferred mode of committing suicide in people with AIDS. In a report of 6 completed suicides from 1990 to 1992 in the Riverside district of London, Pugh, O'Donnell and Catalán (1993) detail the choice of suicide method of these cases. In 4 of the 6 cases described, the people killed themselves by jumping. This is similar to the proportion found by Marzuk in New York. In the past this method has been associated with high psychiatric morbidity, but it is also more associated with men and serious somatic illness. After following a group of both HIV positive and HIV negative drug users, Haastrecht *et al.* (1994) noted that of 7 documented suicides, 5 had done so by violent means. Only 1 person took an overdose. However, 10 other deaths by overdose in the study group may in fact have been carried out with suicidal intent. Others have shown the preponderance of overdose: Pueschel and Heineman (1995) quote 30 per cent and Cote, Biggar and Dannenberg (1992) quote 35 per cent. However, Cote also found an increase in suicides by firearms, and it remained elevated even when adjusted for age and race.

Precipitants

The importance of psychiatric history and previous suicide attempts again appears to predict completed suicide as well as suicidal thoughts and attempts (Pugh, O'Donnell and Catalán, 1993). A past history of DSH was reported in 2 of the 6 suicides described. One of the cases had seen a psychiatrist just four days before the suicide. A similar result was noted in Marzuk's study of New York AIDS suicides. Four of these 12 were known to have had made previous attempts. As most of the studies on suicide completers are conducted retrospectively, information concerning previous psychiatric history is not obtained. It seems that a previous history of self-harm or psychiatric disorder is the best predictor of suicidal behaviour. The Haastrecht study demonstrated that suicidal deaths in injecting drug users did not seem to be related to notification of positive test results; this is a noteworthy finding. Case 6.3 illustrates the unpredictability of suicidal behaviour and highlights the importance of identifying and treating mental illness promptly.

Case 6.3

George was a 33-year-old white gay man who was diagnosed HIV positive in 1988. Since then he had in 1992 been given a CDC3 diagnosis and at the time of initial assessment had a CD4 count of 729. He was initially referred by the HIV service to a psychologist as he was complaining of anxiety and feeling 'paranoid'. After having been seen for a few months, his mental state continued to deteriorate and he was referred for psychiatric opinion.

He denied having any psychiatric problems before going on holiday with a group of friends. He described a sudden change in his mood and at the time thought that someone may have laced his drink with drugs. On returning home, he continued to feel anxious and worried that people were looking at him. He denied any use of illicit substances. However, in recent weeks his mood had become more and more depressed and he also complained about other depressive symptoms.

His appetite was low and he had difficulty sleeping. He described feeling empty inside. One week before this he had taken a small overdose of six paracetamol; he said that he immediately regretted it and confided in his brother, who had been very supportive. He denied current suicidal ideation and said that he felt more secure now that he was receiving help from his friends and family. He was given a diagnosis of major depression, but the aetiology of the paranoid ideation remained in question.

He refused inpatient treatment and, because he was denying current suicidal ideation, he was not thought to be detainable against his will under the Mental Health Act. He was give an antidepressant and a follow-up appointment for the next week. He had arranged to live with his brother in the meantime. Within the week, he had killed himself by a gunshot wound to the head. The coroner's verdict was suicide.

Practical Implications

What can be learned from the research which has already been done? After all, the importance of studying this area is to enable us to identify those at risk of suicide and to prevent the act.

Prevention

There is no single cause of suicidal behaviour but rather a combination of factors. Those at risk will often have immediate problems but may also have more long-standing chronic problems. So how can those most vulnerable be identified in order to prevent an attempt? We have already learned to be aware of personal and environmental risk factors. None of these epidemiological factors represent suicidal intent, which is the essential variable in predicting suicidality. Nevertheless, the presence in an HIV patient of these risk factors should heighten the clinician's concern of suicidality and suggest that a formal suicide assessment needs to be carried out.

Some time periods are high risk intervals for suicide. In the case of HIV there appears to be a bimodal timing at the time of diagnosis and again at the diagnosis of the first AIDS-related illness. In those who have a depressive disorder, the early recovery period is a time of heightened risk. Because of the increased energy and organization seen early in treatment before the mood has had time to lift, the patient may be more likely to act on suicidal thoughts. Bereavement is also a period of increased risk. It can be the source of considerable emotional pain, but the empathy and support which would normally be offered to the bereaved may not be given in a case of HIV because of the stigma still associated with the disease. Also, in HIV, with the ever increasing numbers of those affected, multiple bereavements of friends and partners have become the norm. This further increases the burden on someone who may themselves be infected with the virus. It would seem important, then, to offer support or even counselling to the carers of HIV patients as well as to the patients themselves.

HIV testing in itself can be a harrowing experience. Most fear the outcome of testing and this can be a time when suicidal thinking is prominent. Pre-test counselling attempts to identify those vulnerable and offers accurate information and the opportunity to discuss fears and possible reactions to the result. Questions about suicidality should be a routine part of post-test counselling (Miller, 1995). Often the subject of 'rational suicide' will crop up at different stages of infection. Although this is to be dealt with in another chapter, it is worth emphasizing here the importance of excluding psychiatric disorder, particularly depression. Table 6.3 outlines the psychosocial factors identified in different studies (Sherr, 1995; Rundell *et al.*, 1988; Pueschel and Heinman, 1995). Most important is the existence of psychiatric disorder, particularly depressive disorders and hopelessness.

General measures to reduce the chances of a suicide attempt in someone at risk include making available emergency access to help; identification and adequate management by health and social agencies of those at risk; control of the means used to cause self-harm (in particular, rational prescribing of psychotropic drugs); modification of public attitudes to coping with problems in general and attempted suicide in particular; and measures aimed at improving the material and social circumstances of the population at risk (Hawton and Catalán, 1987).

Table 6.3 *Conditions predisposing to completed suicide in HIV patients*

Psychological factors	Psychiatric factors	Situational factors	Historic factors
HIV coping	Depressive disorder	Relationship issues	History of sexual abuse
Perception of self as victim	Substance misuse	Perceived social isolation	Previous suicide attempt
Fear of AIDS complications	Personality disorder	Bereavement	Past psychiatric illness
Reliance on denial as only defence	Psychosis/schizophrenia	Perceived lack of social support	
Poor judgement and insight		Multiple psychosocial stressors	
Hopelessness		Problems at work	
Loneliness		AIDS-related disease	
Suicidal intent		Separation from partner	
		Waiting for HIV result	

Assessment

Very often clinicians are reluctant to discuss suicide with patients. There is a myth that by asking about suicidal intent, the idea may be implanted in someone who would never have considered it. This is simply not the case. Often it can be a relief for patients to openly discuss their true feelings. Every doctor should be able to assess the risk of suicide. The first requirement is to be prepared to ask directly about the patient's intentions. However, it is not enough to ask bluntly, 'Are you suicidal?' The patient who is feeling hopeless and who longs for death, although has not reached the point of planning the act, may respond 'no' to this question and the opportunity will be missed. Instead, more open questions such as asking how bad the patient is feeling about their situation may encourage them to discuss any feelings of hopelessness or desperation. Others are more secretive about their intention. However, they may offer indirect clues to their intent, perhaps by making frequent reference to death. The question of suicide must therefore be raised with them. Another myth has it that if the patient is saying they are going to kill themself then they are unlikely to do it. In most cases such a warning has been given prior to completing suicide.

In assessing the patient who has presented with some form of self-harm, it is important to gauge the severity of intent. The patient should be asked

Table 6.4 *Assessment of patients after deliberate self-poisoning or self-injury: therapist's questions*

---

1. What is the explanation for the attempt in terms of likely reasons and goals?
2. What was the degree of suicidal intent?
3. Is the patient at risk of suicide now, or is there an immediate risk of further overdose or self-injury?
4. What problems, both acute and chronic, confront the patient? Did a particular event precipitate the attempt?
5. Is the patient psychiatrically ill, and if so, what is the diagnosis and how is this relevant to the attempt?
6. What kind of help would be appropriate, and is the patient willing to accept such help?

Source: Hawton and Catalán (1987).

about any precautions taken against discovery or if there were any warnings given before harming themselves (Table 6.4). Was the intention to die or does the harmful behaviour serve some other purpose such as relieving tension? This may be the case in those with personality disorders. The patient may offer a rationalized explanation for the attempt. It is important to dig a little deeper to look for any other signs that may suggest that the attempt was more serious than they are prepared to admit.

A difficult group are those who repeatedly harm themselves. Unfortunately, the likelihood of suicide is unappreciated by clinicians who assume they have no intention of completing suicide and so take their subsequent attempts less seriously. However, many of them will succeed in killing themselves in the end. It is estimated that 20–25 per cent of chronically suicidal patients eventually kill themselves (Litmun, 1989).

In taking a history, the different problem areas should be identified, including the existence of any of the risk factors mentioned above. The patient should be given time to talk and to discuss their attitudes towards death and suicide. If they have been thinking of suicide, what has prevented them from carrying it out so far? Do they have a good support system at home which may help them through the period of intense suicidality? Whenever possible, family or partners should be interviewed as they may be involved as part of the management of the patient.

Management

How do we help those at risk of suicide? The first task is to decide whether there is serious suicidal risk and if it is associated with psychiatric disorder. If this is so, then the patient requires immediate inpatient psychiatric treatment. Steps should be taken to ensure the patient's safety by removing all dangerous objects, and if necessary, initiate constant observation with one-to-one nursing. If the patient refuses, detention under the Mental Health Act has to be considered.

Usually the suicidal patient can be managed as an outpatient. A prompt psychiatric outpatient appointment should be offered as well as information on how to access the emergency services if the need arises. Treatment will depend on the presence of any psychiatric disorders but in general, if medication is offered, it is also useful to offer supportive psychotherapy which will address some of the problems which have led to the suicidal behaviour.

Dealing with problems in counselling can depend on the stage of infection. In the asymptomatic stage, uncertainty and fears for the future can dominate thinking for some. It can be useful to plan for the future and offer a balanced perspective so they can once again achieve independent living and some hope for the future. In the symptomatic stage, patients will have to deal with periods of bad health and may start to feel hopeless. Helping the patient to see that they have choices and at least some control over their life may help to alleviate this feeling. In the terminal stages, patients can be helped to feel less desperate if adequate palliative care is offered so that they be assured of a dignified death (Miller, 1995).

Summary

There is now a general acceptance that the risk of suicide in the HIV-infected patient is elevated compared to that of the general population. This merits special attention by clinicians who should always be alert to the possibility of suicidal ideation among people with HIV. It is vital that, as part of the evaluation, the clinician attends to signs of hopelessness and enquires specifically about suicidal thoughts or intent. It cannot be assumed that suicide risk is absent if suicidal thinking is simply not mentioned. As HIV infection can result in a wide range of psychopathology and many social stressors, these may be important targets for our prevention strategies.

The evidence suggests there is a greater likelihood that people who become HIV-infected will have other predisposing factors for suicidality. Nevertheless, some attempts seem to be triggered directly as a result of the additional burden of HIV. Some authors have emphasized the specific psychosocial, psychiatric and physical risk factors. It is most likely there is a multiple causality for suicidality in this population (Bellini, 1996).

One finding from these studies which may help us recognize those at risk is the bimodal timing of suicidality. Those thinking of suicide as well as those completing it tend to do so in the early stages after the diagnosis is made and again when they have their first illness. This may help us target our suicide prevention strategies more effectively. The most prominent indicator is the history of previous psychiatric problems and repeated attempts at self-harm. In this respect the HIV patient is not unlike the general population. Also, suicidal thinking is found to be related to chronic physical disease (Belkin *et al.*, 1992).

As long-term survival becomes more likely with the improvements in treatment, there will be more emphasis on quality-of-life issues. HIV-infected patients are living longer, therefore it could be argued that they have longer to consider death. The differing rates of suicide reported in the studies in the last ten years may reflect a downward trend in the suicide rate. However, it is still too early to say if the renewed hope in the new treatments for the virus will result in a change in suicidal behaviour.

References

BECK, A.T., KOVACS, M. and WEISSMAN, A. (1975) 'Hopelessness and suicidal behaviour', *Journal of the American Medical Association*, **234**, pp. 1146–49.

BELKIN, G., FLESHMAN, J.A., STEIN, M., PIETTE, J. and MOR, V. (1992) 'Physical symptoms and depressive symptoms among individuals with HIV infection', *Psychosomatics*, **33**, pp. 416–27.

BELLINI, M. and BRUSCHI, C. (1996) 'HIV infection and suicidality', *Journal of Affective Disorders*, **38**, pp. 153–64.

BROWN, G.R. and RUNDELL, J.R. (1993) 'A prospective study of psychiatric aspects of early HIV disease in women', *General Hospital Psychiatry*, **15**, pp. 139–47.

CARVAJAL, M.J., VICIOSO, C., SANTAMARIA, J.M. and BOSCO, A. (1995) 'AIDS and suicide issues in Spain', *AIDS Care*, **7**, suppl. 2, pp. 135–38.

CATALÁN, J., KLIMES, I., BOND, A., DAY, A., GARROD, A. and RIZZA, C. (1992) 'The psychosocial impact of HIV infection in men with haemophilia', *Journal of Psychosomatic Research*, **36**, pp. 409–16.

CATALÁN, J., SEIJAS, D., LIEF, T., PERGAMI, A. and BURGESS, A. (1995) 'Suicidal behaviour in HIV infection: a case control study of deliberate self harm in people with HIV infection', *Archives of Suicide Research*, **1**, pp. 85–96.

COTE, T.R., BIGGAR, R.J. and DANNENBERG, A.L. (1992) 'Risk of suicide among persons with AIDS', *JAMA*, **268**, 15, pp. 2066–68.

DANNENBERG, A.L., McNEIL, J.G., BRUNDAGE, J.F. and BROOKMEYER, R. (1996) 'Suicide and HIV infection: mortality followup of 4147 HIV-seropositive military service applicants', *JAMA*, **276**, 21, pp. 1743–46.

GALA, C., PERGAMI, A., CATALÁN, J., RICCIO, M., DURBANO, F., MUSICCO, M., BALDEWEG, T. and INVERNIZZI, G. (1992) 'Risk of deliberate self harm and factors associated with suicidal behaviour among asymptomatic individuals with human immunodeficiency virus infection', *Acta Psychiatrica Scandinavia*, **86**, 1, pp. 70–75.

GALA, C., PERGAMI, A., CATALÁN, J., DURBANO, F., MUSICCIO, M., RICCIO, M., BALDEWEG, T. and INVERNIZZI, G. (1993) 'The psychosocial impact of

HIV infection in gay men, drug users and heterosexuals', *British Journal of Psychiatry*, **163**, pp. 651–59.

HAASTRECHT, H.J.A., MIENTJES, G.H.C., VAN DER HOEK, A.J.A.R. and COUTINHO, R.A. (1994) 'Death from suicide and overdose among drug injectors after disclosure of first HIV test result', *AIDS*, **8**, 12, pp. 1721–25.

HAWTON, K. and CATALÁN, J. (1987) *Attempted Suicide*, 2nd edn, Oxford: Oxford University Press.

JAMES, M.E., RUBIN, C.P. and WILLIS, S.E. (1991) 'Drug abuse and psychiatric findings in HIV seropositive pregnant patients', *General Hospital Psychiatry*, **13**, pp. 4–8.

JONES, P. (1995) 'The risk of suicide in people with haemophilia who are HIV infected', *AIDS Care*, **7**, suppl. 2, pp. 157–62.

KIZER, K., GREEN, M., PERKINS, C., DOEBBERT, G. and HUGHES, M. (1988) 'AIDS and suicide in California', *Journal of the American Medical Association*, **260**, p. 1881.

KLEE, H. (1995) 'Drug misuse and suicide: assessing the impact of HIV', *AIDS Care*, **7**, suppl. 2, pp. 145–56.

KONTAXIS, V., MARKIDIS, M., VASLAMATZIS, G., IOANNIDIS, H. and STEFANIS, C. (1988) 'Attempted sucide by jumping: clinical and social features', *Acta Psychiatrica Scandanavia*, **77**, pp. 435–37.

LINEHAN, M. (1986) 'Suicidal people: one population or two?', *Annals of the New York Academy of Science*, **487**, pp. 16–33.

LITMUN, R.E. (1989) 'Long-term treatment of chronically suicidal patients', *Bulletin of the Meninger Clinic*, **53**, pp. 215–28.

MARZUK, P.M. and PERRY, S.W. (1993) 'Suicide and HIV: researchers and clinicians beware', *AIDS Care*, **5**, 4, pp. 387–90.

MARZUK, P.M., TIERNEY, H., TARDIFF, K., GROSS, E.M., MORGAN, E.B., HSU, M.-A. and MANN, J.J. (1988) 'Increased risk of suicide in persons with AIDS', *JAMA*, **259**, 9, pp. 1333–37.

MARZUK, P.M., TARDIFF, K., LEON, A.C., HIRSCH, C.S., HARTWELL, N., PORTERA, M.S. and IQBAL, M.I. (1997) 'HIV seroprevalence among suicide victims in New York City, 1991–1993', *American Journal of Psychiatry*, **154**, *12*, pp. 1720–25.

MILLER, R. (1995) 'Suicide and AIDS: problem identification during counselling', *AIDS Care*, **7**, suppl. 2, pp. 199–205.

O'DOWD, M.A., BIDERMAN, D.J. and MCKEGNEY, F.P. (1993) 'Incidence of suicidality in AIDS and HIV-positive patients attending a psychiatric outpatient program', *Psychosomatics*, **34**, 1, pp. 33–40.

O'DOWD, M.A., MCKEGNEY, F.P., NATALI, C., HARKAVEY, J. and ASNIS, G. (1989) 'A comparison of suicidal behaviours in patients in an AIDS related psychiatric clinic and in a general psychiatric clinic', paper presented at the International Conference on AIDS, 4–9 June (abstract WBP 214)

PATERSON, S.C., VANEZIS, P. and CLAYDON, S.M. (1996) 'Drug addict deaths in north and west London and prevalence of HIV and hepatitis B infection', *Science and Justice*, **36**, 2, pp. 85–88.

PERRY, S., JACOBSBERG, L. and FISHMAN, B. (1990) 'Suicidal ideation and HIV testing', *Journal of the American Medical Association*, **263**, pp. 679–92.

PLOTT, R.T., BENTON, S.D. and WINSLADE, W.J. (1989) 'Suicide of AIDS patients in Texas, a preliminary report', *Texas Medicine*, **85**, pp. 40–43.

PUESCHEL, K. and HEINEMAN, A. (1995) 'HIV and suicide in Hamburg', *AIDS Care*, **7**, suppl. 2, pp. 129–34.

PUGH, K., O'DONNELL, I. and CATALÁN, J. (1993) 'Suicide and HIV disease', *AIDS Care*, **5**, 4, pp. 391–400.

RABKIN, J., WILLIAMS, J., NEUGEBAUER, R., REMEIN, R. and GOETZE, R. (1990) 'Maintenance of hope in HIV spectrum homosexual men', *American Journal of Psychiatry*, **147**, pp. 1322–26.

RABKIN, J.G., REMIEN, R., KATOFF, L. and WILLIAMS, J.B.W. (1993) 'Suicidality in AIDS long-term survivors: what is the evidence?', *AIDS Care*, **5**, 4, pp. 401–12.

ROSENGARD, C. and FOLKMAN, S. (1997) 'Suicidal ideation, bereavment, HIV serostatus and psychological variables in partners of men with AIDS', *AIDS Care*, **9**, 4, pp. 373–84.

RUNDELL, J., THOMASON, J., ZAJAC, R., BEATTY, D. and BOSWELL, R. (1988) 'Psychiatric diagnosis and attempted suicide (AS) in HIV infected USAF personnel', paper presented at the Fourth International Conference on AIDS (abstracts p. 407).

RUNDELL, J.R.L., KYLE, K.M., BROWN, G.R. and THOMASON, J.L. (1992) 'Risk factors for suicide attempts in a human immunodeficiency virus screening program', *Psychosomatics*, **33**, pp. 24–27.

SCHNEIDER, S.G., TAYLOR, S.E., HAMMEN, C., KEMENEY, M. and DUDLEY, J. (1991) 'Factors influencing suicide intent in gay and bisexual suicide ideators: differing models for men with and without human immunodeficiency virus', *Journal of Personality and Social Psychology*, **61**, pp. 776–78.

SHERR, L. (1995) 'Suicide and AIDS: lessons from a casenote audit in London', *AIDS Care*, **7**, suppl. 2, pp. 109–16.

STARACE, F. (1995) 'Epidemiology of suicide among persons with AIDS', *AIDS Care*, **7**, suppl. 2, pp. 123–28.

Chapter 7

Euthanasia, Physician-Assisted Suicide and AIDS

Frans van den Boom, Fabrizio Starace and Erik Hochheimer

Debates about euthanasia (EU) and physician-assisted suicide (PAS) are gaining international momentum. Euthanasia is not, however, something that is specific to AIDS. However, people with AIDS, physicians and researchers fuelled the discussion quite significantly. Although the focus of the chapter is on HIV and AIDS, the broader discussion will be addressed as well. This chapter starts with a definition of different end-of-life medical decisions. Empirical data will be presented for medical decisions involving end of life (MDEL) in general, and for MDEL and HIV/AIDS. The second part of the chapter addresses three recurrent themes with respect to EU/PAS: palliative care and EU/PAS; psychological distress and EU/PAS; (lack of) resources and EU/PAS. Cases will be presented throughout.

Introduction

Euthanasia (EU) and physician-assisted suicide (PAS) are issues that can be looked at from very different angles: the ethical, the religious, the cultural, the utilitarian, the humanistic, the empirical, the individualistic. The fact that this topic can be studied from so many angles makes it fascinating on the one hand, and sometimes frustrating on the other hand. It is like aiming at a moving target. If you've answered some of the questions, someone gets up and tells you that you did not ask the right ones. The following example may illustrate this.

One of the fears surrounding euthanasia and physician-assisted suicide is that decisions with respect to terminating life by means of thanatic drugs are contaminated with inappropriate cost-benefit and budgetary considerations or that vulnerable patients will end their lives involuntarily or succumb to pressure from others to do so. One of the ways to separate fact from fear is to collect empirical data about the amount of time by which life was shortened. If the amount of time is very high, there is reason for caution. Bindels *et al.* (1996) reported that, according to the interviewed physicians, life was not shortened by more than a month in 73% of the persons in the EU/PAS group. The comparative figure for the nationwide study is 91%[1] (Van der Maas *et al.*, 1996). Bindels *et al.* conclude that euthanasia does not shorten life by any significant amount. Furthermore, they state that euthanasia and physician-assisted suicide 'as usually practised' are just 'extreme manifestations of palliation in the ultimate phase of a lethal disease'.

Somerville (1996) opposes such a line of reasoning: 'Bindel's conclusion ... could be taken to imply that the period by which life was shortened is so trifling that it should not be regarded as of any importance. ... It would not be surprising if ... judges or court [sympathetic to arguments that there is a constitutionally protected right to have physician assistance in committing suicide] were to rule, relying on research such as that of Bindels *et al.*, that in a given case the shortening of life by euthanasia was *de minimis* and therefore no crime was committed in carrying out euthanasia'. Then she changes discourses and continues by saying: 'The essence of a case against euthanasia is that it involves one person killing another and that to legalise euthanasia or to institutionalise permission to do it involves the creation of societal symbolism and values that are inherently unacceptable'.

We agree that data as presented by Bindels and Van der Maas should not be used as a basis for decision making about such fundamental issues. However, its value is that it contributes to a demystification surrounding the debate on euthanasia, and such empirical research is needed in order to monitor whether EU/PAS is performed according to the requirements and according to careful medical practice.

Here the emphasis lies on a review of the literature with respect to EU/PAS, accepting the reality of physician-assisted suicide and euthanasia. We do realize that for many people PAS or EU is not a legitimate option for people who are suffering. This rejection of EU/PAS is often in connection with moral, religious and ethical considerations and beliefs. We respect such considerations and beliefs, and have no intention to impose our views on others.

Our position with respect to EU/PAS is that the right of self-determination and the right of personal autonomy, although not absolute, also apply to medical decisions with respect to one's end of life. The principle of self-determination is closely linked to belief in the ability of citizens to make rational and responsible decisions with respect to their health and life, taking into account the freedom, the interests and rights of others (Case 7.1).

Case 7.1

Already some time ago, my brother called me to tell me that he had lost sight in one eye and that he was diagnosed with AIDS. That summer I went to the US to care for him at his home. After a few

---

[1] How reliable are these estimates? It is widely acknowledged that predicting the moment of death is very difficult and hazardous. Both Bindels *et al.*, and Van der Maas *et al.*, use self-report data: the physicians who were involved in performing MDEL themselves estimated the amount of time by which life was shortened.

weeks his physical situation had deteriorated so badly, that he was flown into a hospital. The next evening the treating physician called me and told me that his mental situation had become critical; her diagnosis was AIDS dementia. She euphemistically told me that she was willing 'to help him'. I told her that if it really was AIDS dementia – she had to check on any other possibility – Gerard would want his life ended, but that she was not allowed to administer the drugs until I had arrived. The next day, when I arrived at the hospital, Gerard was lying in his bed, among others linked to a sodium chloride drip, coming back from a pseudo AIDS dementia status. A couple of weeks later he could leave the hospital. Afterwards he came to the Netherlands, and accomplished a few of the things he wanted to accomplish. Less than a year later, again we were taking care of a once vital man, now bedridden, completely blind, Kaposi all over his body and approaching his throat, and suffering from a very nasty neuropathy. His Hb level was so low that he needed a blood transfusion, which he refused, because he did not want his life artificially prolonged. We discussed the possibility of euthanasia once again, and he made clear that if the KS had approached his throat, he wanted his life ended. Two days later he died. No thanatic drugs were administered to him.

This personal story illustrates some of the very difficult issues about end of life decisions. The US experience highlighted three things. Firstly, do not jump to conclusions, check other possibilities first: Gerard had not developed AIDS dementia and in focusing on one hypothesis, his physician had overlooked others. Secondly, this happened in a country where euthanasia still is a criminal offence and physicians are prosecuted if they report what they have done. The situation is still very much the same as 30 years ago, when Glaser and Strauss (1965) described American hospital reality of which euthanasia was part. But this part was hidden and officially denied. When Quill (1994) wrote about him assisting a patient to die, many colleagues said that there was nothing new, except that he had openly written about it. Thirdly, when the physician asked me if I agreed with her 'to help him' I felt a terrible burden: making a decision about someone else's life, even if you've discussed it over and over again, is a terribly sensitive, burdening, emotional and difficult decision.

When Gerard decided that he would not take a blood transfusion, everyone understood why. Prolonging a life he felt was no longer a shadow of life, would have made no sense. But at the same time everyone was relieved that he did not choose the euthanasia option. But if he had wanted euthanasia, we would have walked with him. His physician, my wife, my family and myself. We would have been there to help him face the unknown no matter what happened, and before, during and afterwards we could have talked about it – in the open. (Van den Boom, 1997)

Terminology

Van der Maas and co-workers (Van der Maas, Van Delden and Pijnenborg, 1991; Van der Maas *et al.*, 1996) have distinguished the following medical end-of-life decisions:

- Euthanasia: the administration of drugs with the explicit intention of ending the patient's life, at the patient's explicit request.
- Physician-assisted suicide: the prescription or supplying of drugs with the explicit intention of enabling the patient to end his or her own life.
- Ending of life without an explicit request: the administration of drugs with the explicit intention of ending the patient's life without a concurrent, explicit request by the patient.
- Alleviation of pain and symptoms with opioids: the administration of doses large enough to have a probable life-shortening effect.
- Decision not to treat: the withholding or withdrawal of potentially life-prolonging treatment.

So, whereas in other countries euthanasia has been categorized as active, passive, voluntary and involuntary, in the Dutch definition euthanasia can only be performed if the patient wants it (voluntary) and if a physician acts (active).

Legal Aspects in the Netherlands

The present situation as we know it in the Netherlands did not happen over-night. It took a 30-year discussion and debate. It took courageous physicians, nurses and laypersons to report what they were doing in easing the suffering of patients – remember that EU and PAS have been practised with increasing openness since the 1970s. It took judges that had to create jurisprudence. And it took political will to act upon it.

The present situation in the Netherlands is that euthanasia and physician-assisted suicide are still subject to criminal law (respectively articles 293 and 294 of the Criminal Code). Requirements for accepted practice have been formulated by courts and the medical profession, and in general a physician will not be prosecuted if he or she acts in accordance with the following requirements:

- The patient must consider the suffering unbearable and hopeless.
- The wish to die must be well considered and persistent.
- The request must be voluntary.
- The physician must consult at least one other independent physician.
- The physician may not ascribe the death to natural causes and is obliged to keep records.

Official notification procedures have been established since 1990; here are some of them:

* The doctor performing EU/PAS does not issue a declaration of natural death, but informs the coroner by means of an extensive report conforming to statutory guidelines.
* The coroner reports to the public prosecutor, who decides whether to permit burial or cremation, who examines the coroner's report, and who presents a judgement to the prosecutor general.
* The prosecutor general presents the case, together with his or her own opinion, to the Assembly of Prosecutors General. The assembly provisionally decides whether or not to prosecute. The final decision with regard to prosecution is made by the minister of justice.

On the part of physicians, health lawyers and ethicists, many objections have been expressed against EU/PAS being still subject to criminal law. In 1995 only 41% of all cases of euthanasia were reported (Van der Wal *et al.*, 1996; Van der Maas *et al.*, 1996). In the vast majority of the reported cases, the requirements of careful medical practices were followed. The most important reasons for not reporting were fear, uncertainty and resistance: fear about the general prosecutor undertaking action; uncertainty because it may take more than half a year before physicians are notified if prosecution will follow or not; and resistance because physicians on grounds of principle reject PAS and euthanasia remaining criminal offences (Van der Wal *et al.*, 1996).

On the basis of the second nationwide survey on end-of-life decision making (Van der Maas *et al.*, 1996), the ministers of justice and health proposed another notification procedure. Instead of reporting to the public prosecutor, who reports to the Assembly of Prosecutors General, physicians report to a regional council consisting of the public prosecutor, ethicists and physicians. They judge if the requirements of careful medical practices are followed. If not, the case is passed to the public prosecutor.

Attitudes and Behaviour with Respect to EU/PAS

Doctors

Surveys

Surveys show that between 40% and 90% of physicians have a positive attitude toward euthanasia and physician-assisted suicide (Kenis, 1994). Between 15% and 75% of physicians are in favour of legalizing EU/PAS. Surveys show as well that between 20% and 80% of physicians have been confronted with requests for EU/PAS and that between 5% and 24% have performed it (Table 7.1).

Table 7.1 *Percentage of doctors and nurses who have received requests for EU/PAS and have carried them out*

	Received requests for EU/PAS	Carried out EU/PAS	
Emanuel *et al.* (1996) Oncologists, United States	57.2%	13.6%	
Black *et al.* (1996) Doctors, Washington state	26%	24%	
Lee *et al.* (1996) Doctors, Oregon	21%	7%	
Stevens and Hassan (1994) Doctors, Southeast Australia	33%	19%	
Folker *et al.* (1996) Doctors, Denmark	30%	5%	
Ward and Tate (1994) NHS doctors, United Kingdom	45%	14%	
Hagbin, Streltzer and Danko (1996) Doctors, Hawaii	34%	41%	
Van der Maas *et al.* (1996) Doctors, Netherlands	88%	53%	(ever)
		29%	(last 24 months)
Asch (1996) Nurses, United States	17%	16%	
Leiser *et al.* (1996) Nurses, California	38%	15%	

Differences between Countries

There are significant differences between countries, especially between the Netherlands and the rest of the world. The most plausible explanation is that the Netherlands remains the only country with an official policy on euthanasia. Furthermore, with respect to the high percentage of physicians that are confronted with and performed EU/PAS in the Netherlands, one has to keep in mind that discussing these issues is legitimate in the Netherlands. In the United States and the United Kingdom, the percentage of patients that have had serious thoughts about EU/PAS is much higher than the percentage that have discussed it with their physician. Apparently, the fact that the Netherlands have an open policy, invites patients to bring forward their wishes, resulting in a higher percentage of physicians that have requests for EU or PAS.

Support for Legalization

These surveys demonstrate that a large proportion of physicians support the legalization of physician-assisted suicide. A smaller proportion of physicians, however, are willing to provide such assistance, and an even smaller proportion are willing to inject a lethal dose of medication with the intent of killing a patient (Foley, 1996). This reflects the fact that the North American doctors tend to draw a moral distinction between euthanasia and assisted dying that the Dutch do not. Consequently, in the United States, support for decriminalizing assisted dying has been growing, whereas support for euthanasia remains weak. This difference relates to who is responsible for the final, lethal act: the patient or the physician. In the case of euthanasia, the responsibility lies with the physician; whereas in the case of physician-assisted suicide, the responsibility lies with the patient.

In euthanasia the act of a second person is believed to be morally unacceptable since it is considered equal to murder: 'The essence of a case against euthanasia is that it involves one person killing another' (Somerville, 1996). In PAS it is the patient who determines whether or not they want to continue their life or commit suicide. The conclusion of the Second Circuit Court leaves no doubt: 'In euthanasia one causes the death of another by direct and intentional acts. . . . Euthanasia falls within the definition of murder in New York' (cited in Annas, 1996). In the Netherlands the distinction between EU and PAS is marginal: exactly the same reporting procedures, and requirements for careful medical practice apply. Both with respect to PAS and EU, physicians will be prosecuted only if they have not lived up to the formulated requirements. Interestingly, oncology patients and the general public in the United States make no distinction between euthanasia and physician-assisted suicide (Emanuel *et al.*, 1996).

Covering up Differences

Related to this is the idea that taking PAS and EU together covers up differences in practice. In the Netherlands the number of patients that are assisted in dying is small compared to the number of patients that die after the administration of drugs (Van der Maas *et al.*, 1996). Out of a total of 3,600 cases, assisted dying accounted for 11% (0.2% of all deaths), whereas euthanasia accounted for 89% (2.4% of all deaths). Compared to 1991, the number of cases of euthanasia increased by 900 in the Netherlands. Contrary to expectation, however, the number of assisted deaths remained stable. A possible explanation is that, for practical reasons, physicians prefer EU to PAS. The physician can control a case of euthanasia much better than a case of physician-assisted suicide. More specifically, the physician is in better control with respect to time span between the taking of the drug and the moment of dying. And by acting themselves, physicians can prevent complications (insufficient dose, overdose, vomiting, etc.). The figures in the United States seem to point in exactly the opposite direction: of the 48 oncologists in Emanuel's study that had performed a physician-assisted death or euthanasia, all 48 had assisted in a patient's death but only 6 had performed euthanasia.

Patients

Emanuel *et al.* (1996) reported that in a sample of 155 oncology patients, more than one-quarter had seriously thought about euthanasia and physician-assisted suicide and nearly 12% had seriously discussed these interventions with physicians or others (Table 7.2). In the Netherlands, more than 25% of all people who had died had discussed these interventions, and more than 7% had explicitly requested euthanasia or physician-assisted suicide. Seale and Addington-Hall (1994) report that about one-quarter of respondents and the people who died expressed the view that an earlier death would be preferable or would have been preferable. Some 3.6% were said to have asked for euthanasia during their last year of life.

Table 7.2 *Patients' attitudes towards EU/PAS*

	Serious thoughts	Serious discussion or serious plans	Explicit request	Performed EU/PAS
Emanuel *et al.* (1996) United States, oncology	27.3%	11.9%		
Seale and Addington-Hall (1994) United Kingdom, general	24%		3.6%	
Van der Maas *et al.* (1996) Netherlands, general		25%	7%	2.4%
Green (1995) United Kingdom, HIV/AIDS	33%	19%		
Bindels *et al.* (1996) Netherlands, HIV/AIDS		49%		22%
Van den Boom (1995) Netherlands, HIV/AIDS	66%		25%	23%
Laane (1995) Netherlands, HIV/AIDS				26%
Ogden (1994a,b) Canada, HIV/AIDS	83%	44%		

PAS, Euthanasia and AIDS

The debate on euthanasia is not specific to AIDS, nor was AIDS the starting point of the debate. However, the AIDS epidemic has fuelled the debate quite significantly. It is not coincidental that, next to patients with cancer, recent US jurisprudence with respect to physician-assisted suicide involved patients with AIDS (Annas, 1996; Foley, 1996).

With respect to EU/PAS there are some interesting differences between people suffering from AIDS and people suffering from other illnesses. First, people with AIDS clearly favour policies allowing PAS and AIDS. In a Belgian study, 256 (82%) of people with HIV/AIDS felt that physicians should be able to help terminate the life of an HIV-infected person at their explicit request in the case of severe physical suffering, 158 (50%) in the case of psychological suffering, 81 (26%) simply on demand (Fleerackers *et al.*, 1996). According to Tindall *et al.* (1993), more than 95% expressed support for legalizing EU/PAS. Breitbart, Rosenfelf and Passik (1996) report that 63% of the patients expressed a positive attitude (Table 7.3).

Second, people with AIDS request EU/PAS more often than people suffering from other diseases, and EU/PAS is performed more frequently. A number of studies have been performed in the Netherlands. Van den Boom (1995) reported that about two-thirds of people with HIV had discussed the possibility of euthanasia with their physician, and that 23% died after the administration or taking of drugs with the explicit intention of ending the patient's life. Talking about and making arrangements were a necessary but not sufficient condition for euthanasia. Bindels *et al.* (1996) reported that about half of people with HIV/AIDS had not discussed the possibility of EU/PAS; 22% had died by EU/PAS. Laane (1995) reported 26% as an overall incidence of EU/PAS among people with AIDS in Amsterdam. With respect to other medical decisions concerning the end of life, Bindels *et al.* (1996) reported that they were made in 13% of the cases. Van den Boom *et al.* reported a percentage of 33%. The nationwide study by Van der Maas *et al.* (1996) reported that MDEL have been made in 42% of cases (Van der Maas *et al.*, 1996).

Table 7.3   *People with HIV/AIDS: attitude towards EU/PAS*

	Positive attitude toward EU/PAS
Fleerackers *et al.* (1996) Belgium, HIV/AIDS	82% (severe physical suffering) 50% (psychological suffering) 26% (simply on demand)
Tindall *et al.* (1993) United States, HIV/AIDS	95.2%
Breitbart, Rosenfelf and Passik (1996) United States, HIV/AIDS	63%

In the United Kingdom Green (1995) reported that 33% of the seropositive group (N=57) had considered euthanasia or assisted suicide. This is comparable with the figures of 24% and 28% reported in the cross-sectional study of friends and relatives and those dying from all causes of mortality, excluding sudden deaths (Seale and Addington-Hall, 1994). The illegality of euthanasia clearly affected respondents' attitudes and actions. Eleven of the 19 people with HIV who had considered requesting assistance were planning to hasten death without consultation with, or assistance of, a medical practitioner. In Canada, Ogden (1994a,b) reported that 82% of people with HIV/AIDS had had serious thoughts about EU/PAS, and 44% had had serious discussions about it and had planned for it.

EU/PAS, Relatives and Grief

The study by Van den Boom and co-workers (Van den Boom, Gremmen and Roozenburg, 1991; Van den Boom, 1991) is the only study that looked into the impact of euthanasia and EU/PAS on relatives. In the terminal stage, pleas from relatives did not change the wish to end life by means of euthanasia. Every relative preferred to postpone the act of euthanasia, but respected the patient's decision. No significant association was found between means of death and depression in survivors. However, there is a higher risk for complicated grief if the euthanasia process itself is complicated. In most cases those complications could have been averted, had the responsible physicians been clear about their own moral position right from the beginning or had they had better knowledge about the required dosages of thanatic drugs.

Palliative Care

In many countries palliative care is underdeveloped. One of the reasons most often mentioned is that the focus of Western medicine has always been to cure disease, not to care for people at the end of their lives. Several studies have documented that the care of patients dying in hospitals needs major improvement. In the Support study (Support, 1995) half the physicians did not respect or know about the patient's advance directives; the majority of 'do not resuscitate' orders were not instituted until 24 hours before the patient's death; and most soberingly, 40% of patients had severe and potentially treatable pain for more than several days before they died. Palliative care is needed everywhere, and great educational and organizational efforts are urgently needed to provide it. Promising starts are being made, for example, by removing bureaucratic obstacles to the supply of opioids and training more doctors in palliative care (Case 7.2).

Case 7.2

John is a 39-year-old barkeeper, who lives with his male companion in a spacious apartment. His sister lives on the top floor. John has been suffering from AIDS for three years. A week ago he left hospital in the same condition as he was admitted: a CMV colitis and a non-Hodgkin's lymphoma were making John bedridden and increasingly weak. He had refused chemotherapy, a decision his physicians could easily agree with. John went home to die. His partner and sister would nurse him together with home care around the clock. A hospital bed had been organized. John had discussed euthanasia three years ago, when the diagnosis of AIDS was made after PCP infection. Since then, death or euthanasia had never been mentioned. But now John wanted help: 'This is no life anymore'.

I was asked by my colleague to talk with John. Not in the capacity of 'second doctor' to confirm John's wish. I was asked because my colleague did not feel comfortable about the request. 'It seems John is angry rather than accepting, which I can understand, but still.' I opened the conversation by telling John the exact reason of my visit. Within a minute John talked about his insufficient medication. He wanted more morphine. 'I get morphine twice daily 30 mg, the same as in the hospital. I don't want any pain.' I told John that I would discuss his request with my colleague. That same evening John was given extra morphine. My colleague had been hesitant to raise the morphine because of John's history of drug abuse. He remembered discussing the issue, but was surprised about the importance for John. Three days later John died peacefully in the arms of his partner.

Unfortunately, the lack of palliative and hospice care is often used as an argument against a policy on EU/PAS. Legalization of euthanasia would be not only difficult but also dangerous because it could inhibit the development and provision of adequate palliative care (Foley, 1996). And as the argument continues, this would be disastrous since all suffering can be relieved if caregivers are sufficiently skilful and compassionate, as illustrated by the hospice movement (Cassel and Vladeck, 1996). So with proper palliative care, assisted suicide and euthanasia are no longer needed. Opponents of EU/PAS focus very much on pain relief and symptom management, when making this argument.

There are some comments we would like to make:

- The limited data about patients dying in hospice programs suggests that inadequately relieved pain occurs from 15% to 35% of the time; so at this point it cannot be maintained that all pain can be relieved (Quill, 1994).

- Our treatment of pain is more effective than our treatment of other symptoms such as nausea, vomiting, open wounds and shortness of breath.
- People suffering from pain are not more inclined to euthanasia or physician-assisted suicide. In other words, pain control as part of palliative care is not a substitute for EU/PAS.

The finding of Emanuel *et al.* (1996) that patients experiencing pain were not inclined to EU/PAS is consistent with data from the Netherlands, demonstrating that pain was the only reason for euthanasia in just 10% of cases and a contributing factor in fewer than 50% of cases. Similar results are reported by Seale and Addington-Hall (1994). Although for some, the fear of uncontrollable pain, and fear of controls led to a request for EU/PAS, the overriding concern was about loss of independence and the inability to make personal decisions. Other forms of symptom distress, in the areas of appetite, control, mental functioning, breathing and dependency, show stronger associations with the desire to die sooner and requests for euthanasia. The responses of the people with AIDS in the studies by Ogden and Van den Boom suggest that the decision to plan an assisted death had little to do with a rejection of palliative care or an inability to gain access to quality medical services. Rather it appeared to have more to do with a desire to be in control of one's death – a desire to die in a manner consistent with one's moral beliefs and values, not necessarily with those of the caregiver, as Ogden puts it.

And here are our conclusions:

- 'Though modern palliative methods can ameliorate much of the suffering that accompanies dying, there are still some cases where disintegration and humiliation of the person occurs before death in spite of our best efforts. At the very end of the dying process, even under the watchful eyes of a caring family, supported by a hospice program and a skilled physician, some patients still reach a point where the ravages of diseases make continued living unacceptable. For patients for whom recovery is impossible and for whom further disintegration of the person is all that lies in the future, the motive in choosing death is to preserve what remains of their personhood' (Quill, 1994).
- 'Good comfort care and the availability of PAS and euthanasia are no more mutually exclusive than good cardiologic care and the availability of heart transplantation. Palliative care and EU/PAS stand alongside. The one cannot replace the other' (Angell, 1996).
- Medical decisions that result in the patient's death, whether indirectly by stopping a life-sustaining therapy or by more directly assisting death, should be the intervention of last resort, only after all other possibilities have been thoroughly considered. It seems much more prudent and also much more practicable to establish safeguards against abuse of assisted suicide and euthanasia instead of prohibiting it (Case 7.3).

Case 7.3

Peter is a 40-year-old businessman, who came some years ago to our practice, shortly after he had tested HIV positive. He needed a good general practitioner. To my question about what he thought a good GP meant, he answered straight away that a good GP was someone who was willing to assist in euthanasia. This was extremely important for him, because he was 'the kind of person who needed control over his life, and certainly over his death'. After we had established that both Peter and I had some autonomy here, and that euthanasia was an option, he left. I saw Peter every few months. He was fighting the disease. Every six months I got a report from his AIDS specialist about his CD4, viral load and combination therapy.

However, some months ago Peter was repatriated from his last business trip because of severe neurological symptoms. Peter had a toxoplasma encephalitis. The disease stabilized and he was discharged from the hospital. Friends made some adaptations in his house. His mother, a retired professor of English literature, with whom he had an excellent relationship, came to live with him. Peter could walk a little in his house, but outside he needed a wheelchair. He couldn't write any more with his right hand, something he regretted more than anything else.

Peter made up his mind: 'I have lived fully and I don't want to live like this. I'm going to finish my business, sell my house and that is it'. And he did. He discussed his wish to end his life with his AIDS specialist. I advised Peter to talk to a psychiatrist to exclude any psychopathology. The main reason for this was his life expectancy. Peter was certainly not terminal. We agreed that Peter's wish was valid. We discussed his funeral. I had not seen Peter upset, but the fact that the funeral service only provided coffee and cake, not a lunch for his friends, this made him angry.

Peter died by a physician-assisted suicide at 6.00 pm on a Saturday. His mother, sister and some of his friends were present. When I came at 5.00 pm to give him the barbiturate drink, they were just finishing a banquet. Peter made sure I too had champagne.

Psychological State

A recurrent argument against requests for EU/PAS is that they are a sign of treatable psychological distress, especially depression. Emanuel *et al.* (1996) report that 'oncology patients who were more depressed or who had poor physical functioning were significantly more likely to have discussed euthanasia, to hoard drugs, or to have bought or read *Final Exit* (the Hemlock Society suicide manual)'. They conclude that 'these data, combined with studies on suicidal thoughts among patients with cancer and refusal of life-sustaining treatment among AIDS patients, imply that interest in actions relating to ending of life among patients with life-threatening illnesses are frequently associated with depression and psychological distress'. This conclusion is not supported by the study of Van den Boom (1995):

> We did not find a correlation between arranging for euthanasia and suicidal ideation or suicide. Suicidal ideation was seen more frequently in the group where the stopping and not starting of treatments, and (or) increasing dosages of drugs were prescribed in order to alleviate suffering. It is among the PWAs [people with AIDS] in this group, where depressive and (or) avoidant ways of dealing with the seropositive status and the diagnosis Aids were observed more frequently. It seems that this subgroup is the most vulnerable.
>
> A significant association was found between arranging for euthanasia and better adaptation to the disease. The patients who discussed euthanasia more frequently utilised active behavioural coping mechanisms and more frequently sought social support than patients who had not discussed the option of terminating life by means of thanatic drugs.

The differences between these studies may in part be explained by national differences, and study design. Additionally, differences may be related to the fact that there is a significant disparity between the number of requests for euthanasia and physician-assisted suicide and actually performing it. Hochheimer (1997) reports that an early discussion about the possibility of EU/PAS gives people a sense of control over a situation that is out of their control. In this period, actively finishing life is an option, not a reality. The knowledge that someone is going to be there in case of severe physical and mental suffering, gives them back a sense of control and psychological strength, and opens the possibility to discuss death and dying. As they accommodate to the disease, the need for being in control lessens and is replaced by letting go. This may explain why the majority of people do not want to execute the previously discussed option.

The conclusion, therefore, is not that there is a strong association nor that there is no association. However, the suggestion that all choices in favour of death are irrational, the result of unrecognized and treatable mental illness is absurd and infuriating to those who have spent time at the bedsides of dying patients who are suffering severely with no good choices. The possibility that a request for EU/PAS stems from depressive mood is a legitimate question, but it does not preclude the likelihood that the person is fully rational. Instead of creatively working together to help the patient find death, if that is the only escape, we 'delegitimise the question and sometimes even attack the character or mental health of the struggling patient' (Quill, 1994).

Additional research into the relationship between psychological distress and the request for euthanasia or EU/PAS is needed. It is also necessary to follow up depressed patients to find out whether treatment of depression changes their interest in euthanasia or physician-assisted suicide. Here are several ideas that research should take into account:

- Patients suffering greatly at the end of life may also be depressed, but the depression does not necessarily explain their decision to commit suicide or make it irrational.
- It is not simple to diagnose depression in terminally ill patients. The psychiatrist or psychologist must differentiate appropriate sadness and mourning from major affective disorder which may respond to treatment.
- Remember that terminally ill people can seldom tolerate long-lasting structured interviews, especially if they are under the effects of analgesic narcotics or psychotropic medication.
- In the Netherlands, psychiatrists often participate in the evaluation, but current practice there does not assign a specific role to a psychiatrist or psychologist in certifying that the patient is in sound state of mind and not suffering from depression (a requirement).

Economy

Former US Surgeon General C. Everett Koop stated that in the absence of clear norms and ethics, euthanasia may be determined more by money than by ethical concerns (Koop, 1976, quoted by Ogden, 1994a). In resource-constrained countries, treatments and palliative care are minimal or lacking; in affluent countries a debate about the ceiling of health care expenditures has resulted in proposals not to offer treatment to specific groups (e.g. people older than 65 years, people who have engaged in unhealthy behaviours such as drinking and smoking). Overburdened families or cost-conscious doctors might pressure vulnerable people to request suicide or euthanasia.

One of the fears surrounding euthanasia and physician-assisted suicide is that decisions with respect to terminating life by means of thanatic drugs are contaminated with inappropriate cost-benefit and budgetary considerations, or that vulnerable patients will end their lives involuntarily or succumb to pressure from others to do so. One of the ways to separate fact from fear is to collect data about the amount of time by which life was shortened. If the amount of time is very high, there is reason for caution. Such a finding may indicate that euthanasia and physician-assisted suicide are not end-of-life decisions. Available data point in a different direction; according to Bindels *et al.* (1996) and Van der Maas *et al.* (1996), euthanasia does not shorten life by any significant amount (life was shortened by less than a month in 73% of people with AIDS who died after euthanasia, and in 93% of people suffering from other diseases).

There are three remarks we would like to make:

- Similar wrongdoing is at least as likely in the case of withdrawing life-sustaining treatment. Yet there is no indication of abuse.
- The concern of coercion would hold suffering patients hostage to the deficiencies of our health care system; if the budget is the problem, that problem should be addressed. The euthanasia argument should not be abused to cover up budgetary and distributive problems in health care provision.
- Finally, a question: is it just to 'condemn' a human being to unbearable suffering, in the face of available but unaffordable treatments?

At the Amsterdam International Conference on Home and Community Care, an African man stood up and told us his story and his dilemma. He was a major in the army and relatively wealthy, but he knew that as soon as he developed AIDS, all his savings would disappear, bringing poverty to his wife and children. He very strongly felt that his individual interest counted less than the interest of his family and that his family should be given priority. He considered suicide, was discussing this with his family, and assistance from a physician was very much appreciated by him. What would you do?

Walking the Grey Zone: Concluding Remarks

A request for assisted dying or euthanasia may indicate many things:

- A previously unrecognized mental disorder.
- An unrecognized physical symptom that may be amenable to treatment.
- The patient wants to stop aggressive, burdensome medical therapy, and a hospice approach would now be welcome.
- A family problem, such as caregiver fatigue, that requires a fuller assessment of family coping.
- A spiritual problem as the patient grapples with a god who may be less powerful than previously thought.

And besides all these, there is another possibility:

- A legitimate and rational request for assisted dying by a person who sees his or her situation clearly and has no alternatives that are acceptable (Quill, 1994).

Decisions with respect to physician-assisted suicide and euthanasia are decisions about life and death. It is therefore quite normal, even necessary, that a debate about MDEL addresses the question whether and to what degree man is afforded to intervene in the natural course of dying, and to what degree man is allowed to intervene in life's natural course. On the one hand, medical technology has enabled many diseases to be effectively treated and managed. On the other hand, its prolongation of life has also increased the years of unhealthy existence. And in the terminal stage of our life, a possible negative concomitant of the advanced developments in medical technology is the prolongation of suffering when life is inevitably going to end. 'The increasingly common assertion of a right to determine the time and manner of death . . . represents not only the claim to self-determination, but also a response to the egregious inadequacies and inhumanity that often characterize the care of the dying and critically ill' (Orentlicher, 1996).

But regardless of the available resources, physicians, nurses, other caregivers, patient and relatives will be confronted with medical decision making at the end of a patient's life. At a certain, often undefined point, the quality of death, dying with dignity, becomes the guiding principle of care. The way caregivers respond varies greatly, depending on religious values, moral and ethical values, norms, laws, personal feelings and views, and unfortunately, economic conditions. But caregivers in general and physicians in particular do make decisions with respect to a person who is in a terminal phase of life, or who is suffering from pain and other awkward symptoms: not starting treatment, stopping treatment, pain and symptom relief with or without a foreseen double effect, ending life without an explicit request and ending life with a repeated explicit request. These decisions are difficult and they have to be difficult, because they are the ultimate existential questions, to which there are no simple answers.

References

ANGELL, M. (1996) 'The Surpreme Court and physician-assisted suicide', *New England Journal of Medicine*, **1**, pp. 50–53.

ANNAS, G.J. (1996) 'The promised end – constitutional aspects of physician-assisted suicide', *New England Journal of Medicine*, **9**, pp. 683–87.

ASCH, D.A. (1996) 'The role of critical care nurses in euthanasia and assisted suicide', *New England Journal of Medicine*, **21**, pp. 1374–79.

BLACK, A.L., WALLACE, H., STARKS, H.E. and PEARLMAN, R.A. (1996) 'Physician-assisted suicide and euthanasia in Washington State: patient requests and physician responses', *JAMA*, **275**, pp. 919–25.

BINDELS, P.J., KROL, A., AMEIJDEN, E. VAN, MULDER, D.K.F., VAN DEN HOEK, J.A.R., GRIENSVEN, G.P.J. VAN and COUTINHO, R.A. (1996) 'Euthanasia and physician-assisted suicide in homosexual men with AIDS', *Lancet*, **347**, pp. 499–504.

BREITBART, W., ROSENFELF, B.D. and PASSIK, S.D. (1996) 'Interest in physician-assisted suicide among ambulatory HIV-infected patients', *American Journal of Psychiatry*, **2**, pp. 238–42.

CASSEL, C.K. and VLADECK, B.C. (1996) 'ICD-9 code for palliative or terminal care', *New England Journal of Medicine*, **16**, pp. 1232–34.

EMANUEL, E.J., FAIRCLOUGH, D.L., DANIELS, R. and CLARRIDGE, B.R. (1996) 'Euthanasia and physician-assisted suicide: attitudes and experiences of oncology patients, oncologists, and the public', *Lancet*, **347**, pp. 1805–10.

FLEERACKERS, Y., COLEBUNDERS, R., FONCK, K., DEPRAETERE, K. and PELGROM, J. (1996) 'Euthanasia and physician-assisted suicide', *Lancet*, **347**, p. 1046.

FOLEY, K.M. (1996) 'Competent care for the dying instead of physician-assisted suicide', *New England Journal of Medicine*, **1**, pp. 54–58.

FOLKER, A.P., HOLTUG, N., JENSEN, A.B., KAPPEL, K., NIELSEN, J.K. and NORUP, M. (1996) 'Experiences and attitudes towards end-of-life decisions amongst Danish physicians', *Bioethics*, **10**, pp. 233–49.

GLASER, B.G. and STRAUSS, A.L. (1965) *Awareness of dying*, Chicago IL: Aldine.

GREEN, G. (1995) 'AIDS and euthanasia', *AIDS Care*, suppl. 2, pp. 169–73.

HAGBIN, Z., STRELTZER, J. and DANKO, G.P. (1996) 'Assisted suicide in AIDS: physician attitudes', paper presented at the 149th Meeting of the American Psychiatric Association.

HOCHHEIMER, E. (1997) 'Euthanasia, physician assisted suicide and AIDS in the Netherlands: a GP view', paper presented at the Third International Conference on Home and Community Care for Persons Living with HIV/AIDS, Amsterdam, 21–24 May.

KENIS, Y. (1994) 'Artsen en actieve euthanasie; opinie en praktijk', *Medisch Contact*, **27/28**, pp. 921–24.

KOOP, C.E. (1976) 'The right to die – the moral dilemmas', in Baird, R.M. and Rosenbaum S.E. (eds) *Euthanasia: the moral issues* (1989) Buffalo NY: Prometheus Books, pp. 97–102.

LAANE, H.M. (1995) 'Euthanasia, assisted suicide and AIDS', *AIDS Care*, suppl. 2, pp. 163–67.

LEE, M.A., NELSON, H.D., TILDEN, V.P., GANZINI, L., SCHMIDT, T.A. and TOLLE, S.W. (1996) 'Legalizing assisted suicide – views of physicians in Oregon', *New England Journal of Medicine*, **334**, pp. 410–15.

LEISER, R.J., MITCHELL, T.F., HAHN, J.A. and ABRAMS, D.J. (1996) 'The role of critical care nurses in euthanasia and assisted suicide', *New England Journal of Medicine*, **335**, pp. 972–73.

OGDEN, R. (1994a) *Euthanasia, physician-assisted suicide, and AIDS*, New Westminster BC: Peroglyphics Publishing.

OGDEN, R. (1994b) 'Palliative care and euthanasia: a continuum of care?', *Journal of Palliative Care*, **2**, pp. 82–85.

ORENTLICHER, D. (1996) 'The legalization of physician-assisted suicide', *New England Journal of Medicine*, **19**, pp. 663–67.

QUILL, T. (1994) 'Physician-assisted death: progress or peril', *Suicide and Life-Threatening Behavior*, **4**, pp. 315–25.

SEALE, C. and ADDINGTON-HALL, J. (1994) 'Euthanasia: why people want to die earlier', *Social Science and Medicine*, **5**, pp. 647–54.

SOMERVILLE, M.A. (1996) 'Euthanasia and physician-assisted suicide', *Lancet*, **347**, p. 1046.

STEVENS, C.A. and HASSAN, R. (1994) 'Management of death, dying and euthanasia; attitudes and practices of medical practitioners in South Australia', *Journal of Medical Ethics*, **20**, pp. 41–46.

SUPPORT (1995) 'A controlled trial to improve care for seriously ill hospitalized patients', *JAMA*, **274**, pp. 1591–98.

TINDALL, B., FORDE, S., CARR, A., BARKER, S.T. and COOPER, D.A. (1993) 'Attitudes to euthanasia and assisted suicide in a group of homosexual men with advanced HIV disease', *Journal of Acquired Immunodeficiency Syndrome*, **6**, pp. 1069–70.

VAN DEN BOOM, F. (1995) 'AIDS, euthanasia and grief', *AIDS Care*, suppl. 2, pp. 175–85.

VAN DEN BOOM, F. (1997) 'AIDS, euthanasia and physician assisted suicide', paper presented at the Third AIDS Impact Conference, Melbourne, 22–25 June.

VAN DEN BOOM, F., GREMMEN, T. and ROOZENBURG, H. (1991) *AIDS: Leven na de dood. Nabestaanden over ziekte, dood en rouw*, Utrecht: NcGv.

VAN DER MAAS, P.J., VAN DELDEN, J.J.M. and PIJNENBORG, L. (1991) *Medische beslissingen rond het levenseinde. Het onderzoek van de Commissie Onderzoek Medische Praktijk inzake Euthanasie.* Den Haag: SDU Uitgeverij.

VAN DER MAAS, P.J., VAN DER WAL, G., HAVERKATE, I., DE GRAAFF, C.L., KESTER, J.G.C., ONWUTEAKA-PHILIPSEN, B.D., VAN DER HEIDE, A., BOSMA, J.M. and WILLEMS, D.L. (1996) 'Euthanasia, physician-assisted suicide, and other medical practices involving the end of life in the Netherlands', *New England Journal of Medicine*, **22**, pp. 1699–1705.

VAN DER WAL, G., VAN DER MAAS, P.J., BOSMA, J.M., ONWUTEAKA-PHILIPSEN, B.D., WILLEMS, D.L., HAVERKATE, I. and KOSTENSE, P.J. (1996) 'Evaluation of the notification procedure for physician-assisted death in the Netherlands', *New England Journal of Medicine*, **15**, pp. 1706–11.

WARD, B.J. and TATE, P.A. (1994) 'Attitudes among NHS doctors to requests for euthanasia', *British Medical Journal*, **308**, pp. 1332–34.

Chapter 8

Psychological Interventions

José Catalán

Psychological interventions for people with HIV experiencing psychological difficulties include the use of well-established treatments adapted to their specific needs, as well as the development of novel approaches to deal with their difficulties. Psychological interventions at the time of HIV testing include pre-test discussion and post-test counselling. Interventions for people living with HIV can be psycho-educational, based on community organizations, or more specifically psychotherapeutic, such as problem solving, interpersonal psychotherapy, cognitive-behavioural, psychodynamic, and counselling and supportive psychotherapy. Dealing with bereavement and grief, the development of cognitive impairment, and the problems arising in the context of palliative care can present important challenges.

Introduction

HIV infection can lead to a wide range of mental health problems in individuals living with the infection, and in their partners, relatives and carers, as reviewed in previous chapters. Apart from the treatment of HIV and its complications by means of medical treatments, a variety of mental health interventions can be used to prevent or minimize mental health problems. Such interventions may include the use of medication with effects on mood or behaviour (Chapter 9), and the use of psychological approaches, from counselling to different forms of psychotherapy. Psychological and psychopharmacological interventions are not mutually exclusive, and they can usefully be given at the same time (Markowitz *et al.*, 1998). This chapter reviews the main forms of psychological intervention appropriate for people with HIV.

Organizational Aspects

Mental health specialists working with people who have HIV should not exist in isolation, but rather collaborate closely with the doctors and nurses providing physical care to patients, as well as with social workers, health advisors and others attached to the clinical teams. In HIV care the role of voluntary organizations, non-statutory bodies and non-governmental organizations (NGOs) has been crucial, and in some parts of the world the main task of providing psychosocial support as well as education to reduce the risk of transmission of the infection has been the responsibility of these non-statutory bodies. Again, close collaboration will be needed between NGOs and specialist mental health teams.

Specialist mental health teams involved in HIV care are usually based on the model of the general hospital psychiatric services seen in liaison psychiatry/health psychology, where professionals of various mental health disciplines, such as psychiatry, psychology and psychiatric nursing, work as an integrated team for the assessment and treatment of patients with specific psychiatric problems, as well as for regular meetings and case reviews with doctors and nurses from the medical team (Catalán, Burgess and Klimes, 1995; Royal College of Physicians and Royal College of Psychiatrists, 1995; Clark and Everall, 1997; Pergami and Gonevi, 1997). Unfortunately, such general hospital mental health services are not widespread, not even in developed countries, and there is clear need for services of this kind (Catalán, 1993). Not only do they have a beneficial effect in terms of patient well-being, they also contribute to a reduction in hospital costs (Royal College of Physicians and Royal College of Psychiatrists, 1995).

Recognition of Mental Health Problems

It is clear there is still a strong stigma attached to mental illness, with its association with madness and loss of control, risk of harm to the self and others, and the added implications of weakness and 'lack of moral fibre'. Added to the stigma of HIV infection, it is not surprising to find that both people with the infection and those caring for them may be sometimes reluctant to acknowledge that someone with HIV is also suffering from a mental disorder. Psychological and psychopharmacological interventions can be extremely effective and, contrary to popular but misguided opinion, can contribute to the empowerment and increase in quality of life of people with HIV (Treisman *et al.*, 1994). Attitudes are changing, though, and it is good to see that publications aimed at people living with HIV (Bartlett and Finkbeiner, 1993) promote a positive view of the need to recognize mental health problems, such as depression, and to seek effective help.

There are other obstacles to the recognition of mental health problems in people with HIV. Symptoms such as tiredness, loss of interest in things, headaches or chest pain, could be due both to physical and psychological disorders, and while it is very important to exclude a primarily physical cause for such symptoms, doctors and other may become so blinkered in their need to find a physical explanation, that endless and unnecessary tests are performed, failing to consider the possibility of psychological factors. Alternatively, sadness and tearfulness, for example, may be seen as normal under the circumstances, missing the fact that an understandable psychological response to grief or to fear of death can still be abnormal, in the sense of being out of proportion with the events that cause it or with specific features which suggest more than a simple reaction to threatening events. While sadness or grief are not illnesses, they can certainly be a sign of it, or lead to clinical depression or other mental disorders, hence they require careful assessment.

Assessment of Mental Health Problems

This is not the place to review in detail the conceptual methods and techniques involved in the assessment of possible mental health problems by mental health specialists, such as psychiatrists and psychologists (Catalán, Burgess and Klimes, 1995; Kalichman, 1995; Buhrich and Judd, 1996; Brouillette and Citron, 1997), but it would be relevant here to highlight the reasons for such an assessment, and the need for non-mental health specialists to receive training in mental health issues, and to have access to specialized resources when required.

Commonly, people experiencing psychological difficulties will volunteer their concerns; for example, sadness, inability to cope, panic attacks or insomnia. In some cases, particularly when the person is concerned about the nature of his or her problems, sensitive questioning may be required; for example, with suicidal individuals or those experiencing urges which they regard as unacceptable. Yet in other situations the person may manifest symptoms, such as hyperactivity or elated mood in a manic illness, that the individual does not recognize as abnormal, but which the trained observer would immediately identify as pathological.

Identifying potentially significant symptoms is only the first step. Emotions, thoughts and behaviours will need to be put into context, so their severity, duration, pattern of development and personal meaning can be established. Consider possible reasons for their presence in terms of precipitant factors (what started the problem in the first place), long-term predisposing factors (childhood experiences, early pattern of coping with difficulties), and current maintaining factors (current stresses, unresolved feelings). Detailed clinical assessment and history taking can usefully be applied to the evaluation of depressed mood, suicide risk, psychotic disorders, brain syndromes and personality problems. Standardized instruments can also be of value, such as self-report questionnaires for the assessment of depression and anxiety (Catalán, Burgess and Klimes, 1995; Kalichman, 1995).

By the end of the assessment, it should be possible to have a preliminary formulation regarding the nature and severity of the problems, a preliminary understanding of the factors that contribute to their presence, and an outline of possible forms of help available.

Psychological Interventions at the Time of HIV Testing

HIV Pre-test Discussion

People seeking voluntary HIV testing have higher than expected rates of lifetime psychopathology (Perry *et al.*, 1990; Riccio *et al.*, 1993) and a substantial proportion report suicidal ideas at that stage (Perry, Jacobsberg and Fishman, 1990); these facts highlight the need to make sure the pre-test discussion allows time to help the person clarify the reasons for seeking testing and likely response to the test results. While it is clear that informed consent continues to be necessary and that mandatory testing has been rejected on both practical and ethical grounds (World Health Organization, 1993; Lurie *et al.*, 1994), the recent advances in the treatment of HIV and also in the prevention of transmission to the newborn have made the advantages of knowing the person's HIV status much more obvious, leading to calls for the normalization of the process of HIV antibody testing, within the context of sensitive health care (Miller and Lipman, 1996; Irwin, Valdiserri and Holmberg, 1996; Adcock and Stewart-Moore, 1996).

Post-test Counselling about the Implications of the Result

Breaking the news of the test result, especially a bad result, is likely to require more time and skill than the pre-test discussion, so as to provide sensitive support and accurate information about options that are tailored to the needs of the person at the time, as well as access to further specialist help if needed.

The post-test meeting should aim at dealing with the person's distress, inform him or her about further treatment and ways to remain healthy, and help to prevent the spread of the virus to others. There is evidence that stress prevention training sessions after notification of the test results are the most effective way to reduce distress, regardless of test result, although standard post-test counselling also has some beneficial effects (Perry *et al.*, 1991). Preventive health care to ensure access to the right treatments and preventive strategies can be initiated at this point, although for many this will become a long-term project (Jewett and Hecht, 1993; Rotheram-Borus and Miller, 1998). Risk reduction counselling is appropriate at this time too, regardless of test result. Published evidence, however, suggests that those found to be HIV negative are less likely to modify their sexual behaviour, as reflected in an increase in sexually transmitted diseases in the 6 to 12 months after testing (Zenilman *et al.*, 1992; Otten *et al.*, 1993). There is a debate about the efficacy of interventions to prevent HIV infection, and post-test counselling requires further refining if it is to contribute to preventing infection (Oakley, Fullerton and Holland, 1995).

Psychological Interventions for People Living with HIV

The complexity of the problems created by HIV infection, the characteristics and difficulties experienced by people with the infection, and the social context where HIV occurs mean the provision of effective psychological care for people living with HIV is usually the result of partnership between professional groups, such as medical and nursing teams and mental health specialists; statutory and voluntary organizations; and those working in hospital settings and in the community (Catalán, Burgess and Klimes, 1995; Royal College of Physicians and Royal College of Psychiatrists, 1995).

While there have been few systematic evaluations of psychological interventions in HIV, there is good practical evidence for the value of treatment modalities which have been shown to work in settings other than HIV. Pharmacological treatments for mental health problems in HIV are reviewed elsewhere (Chapter 9).

Psychoeducational Interventions

The changing patterns of treatment response and health outcomes for people living with HIV mean that a long future can be expected for those diagnosed early in the infection, but a future that faces health considerations involving treatment decisions, health maintenance and reduction of risk to others.

Rotheram-Borus and Miller (1998) have developed a model of intervention for young people with HIV based on ethnographic research, which while still largely unevaluated, provides a useful set of guidelines with good face validity. The intervention consists of three modules with a total of 30 sessions which are delivered in interactive small groups. The first module is about *staying healthy* and it includes discussion of attitudes towards living with HIV and future goals, disclosure to others, and involvement in health care decisions and treatment adherence; the second deals with *making sexual decisions and reducing substance misuse*, with emphasis on interpersonal aspects such as discussion of HIV status with potential partners, negotiating safer sex, and handling substance misuse; the third module, *being together*, focuses on identifying goals to achieve quality of life, taking action to maintain quality of life, development of positive routines, and relapse prevention.

The importance of preventive interventions to maintain health in people with HIV has been evident for some time (Jewett and Hecht, 1993), but the development of new effective antiretroviral regimes (HAART) and the importance of a high level of treatment adherence to these drugs has made it particularly important to ensure that people living with HIV taking such drug combinations are well informed about their value and risks, and are given assistance to facilitate treatment compliance. A range of factors can affect treatment adherence (Mehta, Moore and Graham, 1997). San Francisco researchers have outlined the key elements involved in interventions to ensure good treatment adherence, including clarification of the drug regime, development of an individualized plan to integrate the regime into daily activities, self-monitoring procedures, and problem solving for episodes of non-adherence (Chesney and Hecht, 1998).

Support by Community Organizations

The provision of adequate practical support and psychological care for people with HIV infection and their relatives and carers would not have been possible without the developemnt of community organizations and peer support groups, a phenomenon that has taken place both in developing and developed countries (Bartlett and Finkbeiner, 1993; Catalán, Burgess and Klimes, 1995; Brouillette and Citron, 1997). Self-help has been noted as an important factor in quality of life with HIV (Grimes and Coles, 1996), something that community organizations foster. A wide range of help is available, from practical advice and assistance, to counselling for individuals or groups, such as for the newly diagnosed, families with children, or the bereaved. A variety of volunteers, including buddies, can become effective providers of befriending and practical help. Complementary or alternative medicine interventions are usually accessible, including acupuncture, massage and reflexology. While there is very limited research evidence for their efficacy, complementary therapies are very popular, they are perceived as useful by those who receive them, and they are seen as having a place in the comprehensive care needed for people with HIV infection (Catalán, Burgess and Klimes, 1995).

Psychotherapeutic Interventions

A range of 'talking therapies' of general use in non-HIV populations also help people living with HIV. Different theoretical models are used, although a common theme to many of these therapies is that they tend to be short-term, lasting up to six months or so, rather than years, and to focus on the here and now, rather than on childhood experiences.

Problem Solving

Techniques to help people living with HIV to deal with crisis and emotional problems have found understandable favour (Green and McCreaner, 1989), as in the structured training programme described by Fawzy, Namir and Wolcott (1989) to reduce stress and improve coping skills. Problem solving usually involves identifying concerns or problems, prioritizing them in terms of severity or urgency, and then tackling each one in turn by brainstorming and searching for possible solutions, followed by planning how to implement the chosen actions. Further sessions will involve reviewing progress in achieving short-term goals, identifying difficulties or obstacles, and reformulating objectives and agreeing on further steps to be taken. Ideally, problem solving can become a way of thinking and a method to deal with difficulties, regardless of their specific nature.

Interpersonal Psychotherapy

Interpersonal psychotherapy (IP) is a brief, focused psychotherapy for depression; it has been well studied by Klerman *et al.* (1984). Markowitz and co-workers (Markowitz, Klerman and Perry, 1992; Markowitz *et al.*, 1994) have adapted it to the problems of people living with HIV and evaluated its efficacy. IP uses a here-and-now approach, formulates the problems from an interpersonal perspective, and explores changes in four areas of difficulty: grief, role transition, interpersonal disputes and interpersonal deficits. In a controlled study comparing IP with supportive, non-specific psychotherapy for depressed HIV individuals, Markowitz *et al.* (1995) showed greater effects for IP starting after about 8 weeks of treatment and continuing until completion of the 17-week treatment programme. Improvements were apparent in levels of depression as well as in relationships, career and life situation.

A more recent investigation by the same group has further developed these findings. (Markowitz *et al.*, 1998). Depressed people with HIV infection were randomly allocated to one of four 16-week treatment interventions: IP, cognitive-behavioural therapy, supportive psychotherapy alone, and supportive psychotherapy with imipramine, a well-known antidepressant. IP and supportive psychotherapy with imipramine were the most effective treatments in this trial. While there are no reports to date about the value of IP in dealing with the problems arising from the beneficial effects of the new antiretroviral therapies (Chapter 2), this therapeutic approach would seem eminently suited to dealing with problems of normalization, establishing emotional and sexual relationships, and making sense of extended life expectancy.

Cognitive-Behavioural Therapy

The value of cognitive-behavioural therapy (CBT) for a variety of problems such as anxiety and depression is well established (Beck *et al.*, 1979), and there is good evidence for its efficacy for people with HIV-related problems (Catalán, Burgess and Klimes, 1995). Flanagan (1996) has provided a vivid account of its practical use. CBT can be effective in a wide range of problems, from depression and anxiety disorders to more complex difficulties involving long-standing low self-esteem and problems of impulse control, coping difficulties and treatment adherence (Chesney, Folkman and Chambers, 1996; Fukunishi *et al.*, 1997). As with problem-solving techniques, one of the objectives of CBT is to provide the person with a way of thinking and responding to problems, thereby developing a long-term coping approach.

Counselling and Supportive Therapy

There are many different theoretical models of counselling, but they all share a common theme: the provision of a confiding, non-judgemental professional relationship which allows the expresion of painful and distressing feelings, and encourages the adoption of positive coping styles. The need in some cases for culture-specific therapeutic approaches has led to the development of counselling interventions for gay men, drug users, women, people with haemophilia, individuals from ethnic minorities and others (Crawford and Fishman, 1996). Lack of social supports is an important factor in the development of psychological problems, and establishing a confiding and emotionally safe relationship with a professional or with another person with HIV can be of great assistance.

Such long-term support may be particularly valuable for vulnerable individuals with pre-existing difficulties who are prone to cope badly with health problems, social difficulties or emotional turmoil. When depression is present, supportive psychotherapy and antidepressant medication can be particularly effective (Markowitz *et al.*, 1998). Couselling and long-term supportive therapy can include the involvement of partners, children or other relatives, in particular when they are significantly affected by HIV. Counselling may also be very appropiate for individuals attempting to make sense of the impact of new antiretroviral therapies.

Psychodynamic Therapies

Brief focused psychotherapy appears to be effective for non-HIV problems seen in the general hospital (Guthrie *et al.*, 1993), and while there are no comparable studies in patients with HIV, there are some descriptive reports of its use (Milton, 1994; Weiss, 1997). Weiss (1997) has described the value of individual and group psychotherapy for gay men with HIV, identifying the general and specific themes present in this group of individuals. In addition to issues of loss and uncertainty, particular concerns about identity, sexuality and meaning are often seen. In general, psychodynamic interventions may be more appropriate for individuals with long-standing difficulties, usually present before infection with HIV, and who have the capacity to benefit from this form of therapy.

HIV-Specific Psychological Interventions

Breaking Bad News

The issues raised by the breaking of bad news are familiar to all doctors and nurses, but there are particular questions related to the age and background of patients with HIV, their understanding of the condition and their expectations, and the effect of new antiretroviral treatments on survival. These questions will require the professional involved to be well informed and able to answer questions. It is important to provide the information in privacy and without interruptions, attempting to find out first how much the person already knows and how much more needs to be revealed, while responding to the emotional reactions shown by the patient (Buckman, 1993).

Bereavement and Grief

The exposure to multiple losses due to AIDS is one of the especial features of the life of individuals with HIV. Bereavement and grief are normal experiences that can become extreme and sometimes pathological in their duration, severity and characteristics. Several forms of pathological grief have been described: absent or delayed, chronic, inhibited or distorted, severe, and syndromes associated with psychiatric disorder, particularly depression, anxiety and post-traumatic stress disorder (Worden, 1992; Sherr, 1995; Catalán, Burgess and Klimes, 1995).

Most people experiencing normal grief will not seek help from professionals, but a proportion will come into contact with doctors, nurses or others involved in the care of people with HIV. Worden (1992) has described the process of facilitating normal grief, including encouraging the description of events surrounding the death and the expression of related feelings, help to start living without the dead person, providing reassurance about the person's feeelings and reactions, and allowing time to grieve. Voluntary organizations are often able to provide the setting and supports needed to facilitate the process of making sense of loss due to AIDS (Kalichman, 1995; Sherr, 1995).

Grief therapy is appropriate in the case of pathological grief reactions, and here individual crisis intervention approaches have proven effective (Catalán, Burgess and Klimes, 1995). There is interesting preliminary work showing the value of a group-based cognitive behavioural intervention for AIDS-related bereavement (Sikkema *et al.*, 1995).

Palliative Care

The objectives in palliative care are the improvement or maintenance of quality of life, symptom relief and increase in comfort, as opposed to treatment interventions, where remission of disease and treatment of specific syndromes will be the goal, even in the presence of adverse side effects. The end of life can occur in hospital, at home or in hospice. There is some evidence to suggest that in metropolitan areas there may have been a shift away from death in hospital and a trend towards death at home or in hospice, generally reflecting patients' wishes (Guthrie, Nelson and Gazzard, 1996). Apart from pharmacological interventions to control pain, nausea or other undesirable symptoms, a wide range of end-of-life issues may need to be faced, including emotional responses, decision about further care and legal matters, and the response of partner, family and carers (Bartlett and Finkbeiner, 1993; Passik *et al.*, 1995).

HIV-Associated Cognitive Impairment

Many people with HIV infection and their carers become concerned about the risk of HIV dementia. As discussed in Chapter 5, dementia is far less common than originally feared, and there is a possibility that the new antiretroviral treatments may have a further neuroprotective effect (Foudraine *et al.*, 1998). First of all, it is important to ensure that concerned individuals appreciate the nature of the risk, so it is essential to provide acurate and up-to-date information. Typically, individuals afraid of developing dementia are asymptomatics presenting with vague complaints of poor memory and concentration who, after detailed neuropsychological and psychiatric assessment, are found to have normal neuropsychological performance, but to be suffering from anxiety or depression.

In contrast, people with advanced, symptomatic disease and severe immune dysfunction presenting with complaints of impaired memory are often found to be performing poorly on neuropsychological tests. In such cases, as in those of frank dementia, it is important to ensure that information is given to the patient in a way that can be understood, and that help is given to the person with HIV and to his or her carers and relatives about the implications of the diagnosis. Practical decisions about property and legal matters, as well as concerning further medical and social care will need to be made, and the person with HIV will usually wish to be involved.

References

ADCOCK, J. and STEWART-MOORE, J. (1996) 'Pre-test-counselling for HIV', *British Journal of Midwifery*, **4**, pp. 196–98.

BARTLETT, J.G. and FINKBEINER, A.K. (1993) *The Guide to Living with HIV Infection*, London: Johns Hopkins University Press.

BECK, A.T., RUSH, J.A., SHAW, B.F. *et al.* (1979) *Cognitive treatment of depression*, New York: Guilford.

BROUILLETTE, M.J. and CITRON, K. (1997) *HIV and Psychiatry: a training and resource manual*, Ottawa: Canadian Psychiatric Association.

BUCKMAN, R. (1993) 'Communications in palliative care', in Doyle, D., Hanks, G. and MacDonald, N. (eds) *Oxford Textbook of Palliative Medicine*, Oxford: Oxford University Press.

BUHRICH, N. and JUDD, F.K. (1996) 'HIV and psychiatric disorders', *Medical Journal of Australia*, **164**, pp. 422–24.

CATALÁN, J. (1993) *HIV infection and mental health care: implications for services*, Copenhagen: WHO European Office.

CATALÁN, J., BURGESS, A. and KLIMES, I. (1995) *Psychological Medicine of HIV infection*, Oxford: Oxford University Press.

CHESNEY, M. and HECHT, F. (1998) 'Adherence to HIV antiretroviral therapy: an essential element to understanding treatment effect', paper presented at the Second European Conference on the Methods and Results of Social and Behavioural Research on AIDS, Paris, 12–15 January.

CHESNEY, M., FOLKMAN, S. and CHAMBERS, D. (1996) 'Coping effectiveness training for men living with HIV: preliminary findings', *International Journal of STD and AIDS*, **7**, pp. 75–82.

CLARK, B.R. and EVERALL, I.P. (1997) 'What is the role of the HIV liaison psychiatrist?' *Genitourinary Medicine*, **73**, pp. 568–70.

CRAWFORD, I. and FISHMAN, B. (eds) (1996) *Psychosocial Interventions in HIV Disease*, London: Jason Aronson.

FAWZY, F.I., NAMIR, S. and WOLCOTT, D.L. (1989) 'Structured group intervention model for AIDS patients', *Psychiatric Medicine*, **7**, pp. 35–45.

FLANAGAN, C. (1996) 'Cognitive-behavioural treatment strategies for emotionally distressed asymptomatic seropositives', in Crawford, I. and Fishman, B. (eds) *Psychosocial Interventions in HIV Disease*, London: Jason Aronson.

FOUDRAINE, N., HOETELMANS, R., LANGE, J. *et al.* (1998) 'Cerebrospinal-fluid HIV 1 RNA and drug concentrations after treatment wih lamivudine plus zidovudine or stavudine', *Lancet*, **351**, pp. 1547–51.

FUKUNISHI, I., HOSAKA, T., MATSUMOTO, T. *et al.* (1997) 'Liaison psychiatry and HIV infection II: application of relaxation in HIV positive patients', *Psychiatry and Clinical Neurosciences*, **51**, pp. 5–8.

GREEN, J. and MCCREANER, A. (1989) *Counselling in HIV infection and AIDS*, Oxford: Blackwell Scientific.

GRIMES, D.E. and COLES, F.L. (1996) 'Self-help and life quality in persons with HIV disease', *AIDS Care*, **8**, pp. 691–99.

GUTHRIE, B., NELSON, M. and GAZZARD, B. (1996) 'Are people with HIV in London able to die where they plan?', *AIDS Care*, **8**, pp. 709–13.

GUTHRIE, E., CREED, F., DAWSON, D. *et al.* (1993) 'A randomized controlled trial of psychotherapy in patients with refractory irritable bowel syndrome', *British Journal of Psychiatry*, **163**, pp. 315–21.

IRWIN, K.L., VALDISERRI, R.O. and HOLMBERG, S.D. (1996) 'The acceptability of voluntary HIV antibody testing in the US: a decade of lessons learned', *AIDS*, **10**, pp. 1707–17.

JEWETT, J.F. and HECHT, F.M. (1993) 'Preventive health care for adults with HIV infection', *Journal of the American Medical Association,* **269**, pp. 1144–53.

KALICHMAN, S.C. (1995) *Understanding AIDS: a guide for mental health professionals*, Washington DC: American Psychological Association.

KLERMAN, G.L., WEISSMAN, M.M., ROUNSAVILLE, B.J. *et al.* (1984) *Interpersonal psychotherapy for depression*, New York: Basic Books.

LURIE, P., AVINS, A., PHILLIPS, K. *et al.* (1994) 'The cost-effectiveness of voluntary counselling and testing of hospital inpatients for HIV infection', *Journal of the American Medical Association*, **272**, pp. 1832–38.

MARKOWITZ, J., KLERMAN, G. and PERRY, S. (1992) 'Interpersonal psychotherapy of depressed HIV-positive outpatients', *Hospital and Community Psychiatry*, **43**, pp. 885–90.

MARKOWITZ, J., KLERMAN, G., PERRY, S. *et al.* (1994) 'Interpersonal psychotherapy for depressed HIV-seropositive patients', in Klerman, G. and Weissman, M. (eds) *New Applications of Interpersonal Psychotherapy*, Washington DC: American Psychiatric Press.

MARKOWITZ, J., KLERMAN, G., CLOUGHERTY, K. *et al.* (1995) 'Individual psychotherapies for depressed HIV-positive patients', *American Journal of Psychiatry*, **152**, pp. 1504–9.

MARKOWITZ, J., KOCSIS, J., FISHMAN, B. *et al.* (1998) 'Treatment of depressive symptoms in HIV positive patients', *Archives of General Psychiatry*, **55**, pp. 452–57.

MEHTA, S., MOORE, R. and GRAHAM, N. (1997) 'Potential factors affecting adherence with HIV therapy', *AIDS*, **11**, pp. 1665–70.

MILLER, R. and LIPMAN, M. (1996) 'HIV pre-test discussion', *British Medical Journal*, **313**, p. 130.

MILTON, M. (1994) 'The case for existential therapy in HIV-related psychotherapy', *Counselling Psychology Quarterly*, **7**, pp. 367–74.

OTTEN, M.W., ZAIDI, A.A., WROTEN, J. *et al.* (1993) 'Changes in sexually transmitted disease rates after HIV testing and post-test counselling', *American Journal of Public Health*, **83**, pp. 529–33.

PASSIK, S.D., MCDONALD, M.V., ROSENFELD, B.D. *et al.* (1995) 'End of life issues in patients with AIDS: clinical and research considerations', *Journal of Pharmaceutical Care in Pain and Symptom Control*, **3**, pp. 91–111.

PERGAMI, A. and GONEVI, M. (1997) 'A biopsychosocial approach to the mental health aspects of HIV disease', *Italian Journal of Psychiatry and Behavioural Sciences*, **3**, pp. 107–9.

PERRY, S.W., JACOBSBERG, L. and FISHMAN, B. (1990) 'Suicidal ideation and HIV testing', *Journal of the American Medical Association*, **263**, pp. 679–82.

PERRY, S.W., JACOBSBERG, L., FISHMAN, B. *et al.* (1990) 'Psychiatric diagnosis before serological testing for HIV', *American Journal of Psychiatry*, **147**, pp. 89–93.

PERRY, S.W., FISHMAN, B., JACOBSBERG, L. *et al.* (1991) 'Effectiveness of psychoeducational intervention in reducing emotional distress after HIV antibody testing', *Archives of General Psychiatry*, **48**, pp. 143–47.

RICCIO, M., PUGH, K., JADRESIC, D. *et al.* (1993) 'Neuropsychiatric aspects of HIV-1 infection in gay men: controlled investigation of psychiatric, neuropsychological and neurological status', *Journal of Psychosomatic Research*, **17**, pp. 819–30.

ROTHERHAM-BORUS, M.J. and MILLER, S. (1998) 'Secondary prevention for youths living with HIV', *AIDS Care*, **10**, pp. 17–34.

Royal College of Physicians and Royal College of Psychiatrists (1995) *The Psychological Care of Medical Patients*, London: Royal College of Physicians and Royal College of Psychiatrists.

SHERR, L. (ed.) (1995) *Grief and AIDS*, Chichester: John Wiley.

SIKKEMA, K.J., KALICHMAN, S.C., KELLY, J.A. *et al.* (1995) 'Group intervention to improve coping with AIDS-related bereavement: model development and an illustrative clinical example', *AIDS Care*, **7**, pp. 463–73.

TREISMAN, G., FISHMAN, M., LYKETSOS, C. *et al.* (1994) 'Evaluation and treatment of psychiatric disorders associated with HIV infection', in Price, R.W. and Perry, S.W. (eds) *HIV, AIDS and the brain*, New York: Raven Press.

WEISS, J.J. (1997) 'Psychotherapy with HIV-positive gay men: a psychodynamic perspective', *American Journal of Psychotherapy*, **51**, pp. 31–44.

WORDEN, J.W. (1992) *Grief counselling and grief therapy: a handbook for the mental health practitioner*, London: Routledge.

WORLD HEALTH ORGANIZATION (1993) *Statement from the consultation on testing and counselling for HIV infection.* Geneva: WHO Global Programme on AIDS.

ZENILMAN, J.M., ERICKSON, B., FOX, R. *et al.* (1992) 'Effect of HIV posttest counselling on STD incidence', *Journal of the American Medical Association*, **267**, pp. 843–45.

Chapter 9

Psychopharmacological Treatments

Ashok N. Singh and José Luis Ayuso Mateos

The purpose of all drug therapy is clinical efficacy. As a practical matter, this requires the delivery of the right drug to the right place in the right concentration for the right amount of time. Most guidelines available to the clinicain for the psychopharmacological managment of psychiatric patients are derived from studies of medically well patient populations; these guidelines may not be reliable for the individual patients in whom pharmacokinetic changes are large enough to require alterations in drug dosages. One factor among many that may produce these changes is medical illness. HIV-related problems are present in most medical specialities, and psychiatry has not been spared. The use of psychotropic medication in patients with HIV infection can be challenging, and the psychiatrist must confront a series of problems when considering the prescription of psychotropics to HIV-infected patients, especially the coexistence of multiple medical illnesses, the concomittent use of other medications, and the absence of specific guidelines. This chapter summarizes the general guidelines for use of psychopharmacological medication in this group of patients.

Depression

Heterocyclic Antidepressants

Tricyclic antidepressants have proven effective in treating depressed HIV-positive patients in both controlled (Manning *et al.*, 1990; Rabkin *et al.*, 1994) and open clinical studies (Rabkin and Harrison, 1990; Fernandez and Levy, 1991). HIV-infected patients are similar to geriatric patients in their response to the administration of antidepressants. They can respond to lower dosages of tricyclics (25–100 mg), but they may also suffer severe anticholinergic effects at reduced dosages. Therefore, the choice of an antidepressant for these patients should be guided, by its side effects profile. The administration of agents with a high affinity for central muscarine receptors should be avoided, since their anticholinergic effects could aggravate cognitive difficulties to the point of triggering delirium episodes. In addition, they produce dryness in the mucous membranes, which could favour the development of candidiasis. Due to its milder side effects on the autonomic nervous system, nortriptyline is a useful drug here.

Patients in the advanced stages of AIDS have a lower tolerance for tricyclics and do not respond to them as well. Some authors recommend the use of tricyclic agents in asymptomatic HIV-infected patients and in AIDS patients who have neither a systematic illness nor significant cognitive deterioration (Ochitill, 1992).

In physically symptomatic HIV patients, initial dosages are usually one-fourth to one-half of those used in other psychiatric patients (e.g. nortriptyline at 10 mg daily). The most frequent side effects with these antidepressants are the same as in non-HIV patients (dry mouth, agitation or sedation, urinary retention, constipation), although they are likely to be of a greater magnitude in AIDS patients. In patients with significant diarrhoea and/or long-standing insomnia, the side effects of tricyclics may actually alleviate these problems.

Monoamine Oxidase Inhibitors

A review of the literature failed to provide data regarding the use of monoamine oxidase inhibitors (MAOIs) in HIV-infected individuals. The dietary restrictions which accompany treatment with these agents could exacerbate the nutritional problems associated with HIV-infection. And there is a need to be even more cautious with patients who are simultaneously taking MAOIs and zidovudine (AZT), since AZT has an inhibiting effect on the enzyme catecholamine *o*-methyl transferase (Fernandez and Levy, 1990). Another interaction which should be kept in mind when using MAOIs is with sulphonamides. Their simultaneous use could set off an increase in the plasmatic levels of both agents (Ochitill, 1992).

SSRIs

The new selective serotonin reuptake inhibitors (SSRIs) appear to be of comparable efficacy to the older preparations in treating depression, and possibly feature a better side effects profile, although they are currently much more expensive. Many clinicians prefer the newer drugs in the medically ill, not only because of their higher acceptance among patients, but also because of their greater safety margin in overdose.

Fluoxetine

Open studies have been published showing therapeutic responses to fluoxetine (Levine *et al.*, 1990; Perkins *et al.*, 1991). Its side effects in these cases were transient and minimal, including mild anxiety, insomnia, and gastrointestinal discomfort, but no weight loss. In an open treatment study, fluoxetine alone and fluoxetine plus dextroamphetamine were found to be effective treatments for patients with HIV and depression who did not experience persistent improvement on imipramine, regardless of the initial level of immune deficiency or number or type of HIV medications used concurrently. No negative effects on immune status were observed with treatment (Rabkin, Rabkin and Wagner, 1994).

In an open study of fluoxetine compared with bupropion (Ochitill, 1992) in patients with secondary depression (depression which appeared after or at the same time as the HIV infection), a marked or moderate therapeutic response was reported in 66 per cent, of the subjects who had major depression, and in 72 per cent, of those who had an organic affective disorder.

In symptomatic patients, initial dosages with fluoxetine should be low (10 mg daily). During the first few weeks of treatment, fluoxetine can cause restlessness, insomnia, agitation or gastrointestinal, disturbances, which then tend to cease, a phenomenon also observed in HIV negative individuals. Weight loss during treatment with this agent, which is seen in depressed patients not suffering from an organic pathology, should be kept in mind when prescribing it to AIDS patients in advanced stages, since they frequently show signs of malnourishment and anorexia. An uncommonly observed side effect of fluoxetine relevant to this group of patients is the possibility of inducing akathisia, which has been related to its potent serotonergic activity (Lipinski *et al.*, 1989).

In using this medication, the physician must take into account the long half-life of fluoxetine and its principal metabolite, norfluoxetine, as well as the dependence of its metabolism on hepatic activity. Simultaneous prescription of medication which interferes with hepatic metabolism can set off an increase in plasmatic levels, even to the point of toxicity (Fuller *et al.*, 1989). These agents include tricyclics, neuroleptics, anticonvulsants, beta blockers, and some benzodiazepines.

Sertraline

In an open trial with sertraline at an initial dosage of 50 mg/day, increased as needed up to a maximum of 200 mg/day, it was shown that this drug was an effective, well-tolerated treatment for depression which presented no apparent adverse effects on immune status (Rabkin, Wagner, and Rabkin, 1994). Concurrently administered drugs included acyclovir, AZT and sulphamethoxazole, fluconazole, pentamidine and dapsone. There were no interactions reported in this study. The advantages of sertraline over other serotonergic agents, such as fluoxetine, include its shorter half-life (26 hours compared with 2–3 days for fluoxetine).

Paroxetine

In the published clinical trials involving these SSRIs, in a reduced number of cases a good response has been observed at dosages of 20 mg/day of paroxetine in depressed HIV-infected patients (Singh and Catalán, 1996). A significant percentage of the subjects who received this agent reported erectile dysfunction as a side effect. This dysfunction can be succesfully treated by yohimbine (Singh, Scurlock and Catalán, 1995).

Bupropion

Reports have also been published regarding the efficacy of new antidepressants, such as bupropion, in the treatment of depression in HIV-infected patients. In an open study, bupropion seemed superior to fluoxetine in improving anhedonic patients, but there was a high inicidence of patients on bupropion developing convulsions when their dosage was raised above 300 mg/day (Ochitill, 1992). This adverse side effect also appeared in patients suffering from an organic mental disorder. These authors' experiences indicate the need to take strict precautions when bupropion is administered to neurologically compromised patients, using a fixed dosage distributed in three or four daily doses.

Other Agents

Testosterone

A recent report presents the effect on depressed mood of testosterone replacement therapy in HIV positive men with significant immunosupression and clinically low levels of serum testosterone (Rabkin and Rabkin, 1995). The open trial consisted of intramuscular (i.m.) injection of testosterone propionate every other week at doses of 200–400 mg, in a sample comprising 26 subjects with significant mood problems, defined by Hamilton depression scale scores of 14 or more. In 69 per cent of the patients an improvement in mood was observed at the end of 8 weeks of treatment. However, although these results are promising, it must be remembered that this was merely a preliminary report, and that only 29 per cent of the subjects met DSM IIIR criteria for major depression and dysthymia.

L-Acetylcarnitine

L-Acetylcarnitine is a natural isomer of a substance present in the brain, and structurally related to acetycholine. A double-blind study against placebo showed that, at dosages of 500 mg/day, this substance significantly reduced anxious and depressive symptoms in HIV-infected patients (De Simone *et al.*, 1988).

Psychostimulants

Stimulants, such as methylphenidate and dextroamphetamine, can improve mood and attention and lead to increase in energy, and they have been used in the treatment of depressive disorders in the medically ill (Chiarello and Cole, 1987; Kauffman *et al.*, 1989). There are no controlled investigations of the value of psychostimulants in HIV infection, although uncontrolled studies in depressed people with HIV infection who had not responded to tricyclic antidepressant with some degree of cognitive impairment, these have shown improvement in mood and cognitive functioning (Fernandez, Adams and Levy, 1988). And Wagner, Rabkin and Rabkin (1997), concluded that dextroamphetamine is a potentially effective and fast-acting antidepressant treatment for this population. Psychostimulants tend to be used for short periods of time, often during the terminal phase of the illness. The lack of controlled studies and their possible side effects (agitation, elated mood, restlesness, anorexia and weight loss, paranoid syndromes and risk of misuse) means that if they are to be prescribed, it should be under close monitoring and evaluation.

Psychosis

Psychotic disorders, such as mania and schizophrenia, can occur in people with HIV infection. In some cases the psychotic symptoms may be the result of subtle or gross brain pathology associated with HIV infection, while in others it may be iatrogenic (steroids) or secondary to substance misuse (World Health Organization, 1990; McGowan *et al.*, 1991). Recent publications have also indicated that psychiatric patients may be considered a group at risk for contracting HIV infection (Stefan and Catalán, 1995; Ayuso Mateos *et al.*, 1997).

Antipsychotics

Neuroleptics are the treatment of choice for the proper control of psychotic symptoms. They are also widely prescribed for the management of delirium episodes, heightening the analgesic effects of narcotics, and treating nausea.

The risk of developing antipsychotic-induced extrapyramidal symptoms (EPS) is 2–4 times higher in psychotic AIDS patients than in psychotic patients without AIDS (Hriso, Kuhn and Maslev, 1991). However, when evaluating these neurological effects, it is important to remember that 11 per cent of AIDS patients who present neurological complications have abnormal movements without exposure to dopaminergic antagonists (Nath, Janckovic and Pattigrew, 1987). It has also been suggested that this population may have an increased risk of developing tardive dyskinesia (Shedlack, Soldato-Couture and Swanson, 1994).

Among the severe side effects related to the administration of antipsychotics which have been described in the literature, one of the most striking is the development of neuroleptic malignant syndrome (Burch and Montoya, 1989) and severe dystonic reactions (Halstead *et al.*, 1988) observed both with incisive neuroleptics, such as haloperidol, and with others of lesser potency, such as chlorpromazine. Published descriptions of neuroleptic malignant syndrome (NMS) indicate that it appears between 36 hours and 12 weeks after the beginning of treatment with moderate dosages of neuroleptics. In addition, NMS has been described with agents having a low affinity for dopaminergic receptors, such as prochlorperazine (Bernstein and Scherokmon, 1986). A reappearance of NMS upon reinstating neuroleptic treatment, whether with the same agent or a different one, has also been described (Breitbart, Marotta and Call, 1988). The presence of organic cerebral deterioration, in particular HIV-associated dementia, is a risk factor for the development of NMS.

Some clinicians have reported a lower incidence of severe extrapyramidal reactions in patients treated with molindone or thioridazine to control their psychotic symptoms, as compared to those treated with haloperidol (Fernandez and Levy, 1993; Harris, Jeste and Gledhorn, 1991). Some of the patients respond to low dosages of neuroleptics, approximately 1–5 mg of haloperidol twice a day or an equivalent dosage of incisive neuroleptics (Ostrow, Grant and Atkinson, 1988). In those patients with schizophrenic psychosis who are also HIV-infected, the necessary dosages are similar to those used for other schizophrenic patients, although there seems to be an increase in side effects from neuroleptics as the illness progresses. The progressive drop in body mass in its more advanced stages should also be considered, in order to adjust the dosage accordingly.

In HIV-infected patients, above all those in an advanced stage of the illness or who are receiving other drugs that have effects on the cardiovascular system, it is important to keep in mind the side effects due to alpha-adrenergic blockage produced by low potency neuroleptics, side effects such as orthostatic hypotension or tachycardia. Chlorpromazine also has a negative inotropic effect.

In general, when using neuroleptics in this population, the best course is to start off with low doses of incisive neuroleptics, and increase the dosage slowly and progressively. Given the frequent affectation of the central nervous system in these patients, and their susceptibility to delirium, the initial use of anti-Parkinsonian correctors is not indicated. If extrapyramidal symptoms arise, the physician must either add correcting medication or change to a sedative neuroleptic. Bromperidol has been used in brain-damaged patients exhibiting psychotic symptoms, with good results (Peretta *et al.*, 1992).

The new atypical antipsychotic, remoxipride, a selective dopamine D2 antagonist, has been used with good results, but in view of its possible contribution to aplastic anaemia, remoxipride should be used with caution (Scurlock, Singh and Catalán, 1995). A newer antipsychotic, risperidone, a 5-HT2/dopamine D2 antagonist, has been associated with fewer extrapyramidal side effects and used successfully in this group of patients (Singh and Catalán, 1994; Singh, Galledge and Catalán, 1997). Clozapine can produce undesirable haematological effects, centred on the appearance of agranulocitosis. We do not believe that its use is appropriate in HIV-infected patients, since they can also present haematologic abnormalities as a consequence of antiretroviral treatment and/or systemic illness.

Lithium and Anticonvulsants

Lithium is indicated in those patients who were receiving it for an affective disorder which appeared before their HIV infection. It is also effective in the management of manic syndromes related to AZT therapy. When administering lithium to these patients, it is important to exercise extreme caution, due to the frequent development of episodes of diarrhoea in AIDS patients.

Immunosuppressed HIV-infected patients tolerate neuroleptics and lithium poorly (Halman *et al.*, 1993). In these situations, anticonvulsant medication (carbamazepine, sodium valproate) can adequately control the acute symptoms of a manic episode. The administration of carbamazepine should include strict control of these patients' haemopoietic function, above all because they are frequently taken with other drugs, such as AZT, which can also trigger toxic effects in the bone marrow.

Anxiety and Insomnia

Psychological interventions are the treatment of choice for anxiety disorders and insomnia, and the use of long-term anxiolytic medication should not be encouraged. In general, it is best to prescribe anxiolytics for a limited period of time, while other psychological and social interventions are introduced. The routine administration of hypnotic medication should be avoided in AIDS patients. Clinicians should begin by employing non-pharmacological sleep-enhancing measures and by relieving physical symptoms, such as pain, which could be responsible for the patient's insomnia (Ochitill, 1992).

Studies on the interactions between benzodiazepines and the medication habitually used in AIDS treatment are scarce. The pharmacokinetics of oxazepam in combination with AZT has been evaluated, without finding variations in the plasmatic levels of either agent when they were used together, although the side effect of headaches was more common in patients taking both of them at once (Male *et al.*, 1992). The simultaneous administration of benzodiazepines and ketoconazole or isoniazide produces a slight increase in the benzodiazepine level; whereas the administration of these anxiolytic agents and rifampicin moderately decreases the benzodiazepine level (Trachman, 1992).

Because of their potential for abuse and the side effects detailed above, some investigators have proposed buspirone as an alternative in HIV-infected patients who are addicted to opiates (Batki, 1990). But remember that buspirone has a direct agonistic effect due to its affinity for dopaminergic presynaptic receptors, and can worsen extrapyramidal symptoms (Brody *et al.*, 1990). A case of buspirone-induced psychosis has been described in an HIV-infected patient. The appearance of such a clinical syndrome could be related to this agent's dopaminergic effect (Trachman, 1992). Antidepressant drugs can also be used to treat anxiety disorders, particularly those with phobic obsessional symptoms.

Delirium

Delirium is one of the organic mental disorders observed most frequently in hospitalized HIV-infected patients (Wolcott, Fawzy and Pasnau, 1985; Ayuso *et al.*, 1989). A conservative attitude has been recommended for the management of these conditions, with the use of low oral or intramuscular doses of neuroleptics, and correction of the organic disorders responsible for the development of disturbances in the level of consciousness (Breitbart *et al.*, 1996). Other authors have postulated that patients suffering from delirium and agitation should be given high doses of neuroleptics, alone or in combination with lorazepam, in cases where quick control of the symptoms is vital (Fernandez *et al.*, 1989).

In general, the delirium symptoms which appear in HIV patients, above all when there is overlapping dementia, respond to low dosages of neuroleptics – 2.5 mg/day of haloperidol, 50 mg/day of chlorpromazine (Sidtis *et al.*, 1993). The fact they respond to such low dosages can be explained by the altered pharmacokinetics of subjects who are severely organically compromised, and by the alterations in the subcortical structures mentioned above. In other populations of weakened patients, e.g. patients suffering from cancer or geriatric patients, a good response in delirium symptoms has also been observed with low dosages of antipsychotics. The efficacy of pharmacological interventions in patients with delirium is increased if they take place as soon as the first symptoms appear.

The use of benzodiazepines, such as lorazepam, for the management of these conditions is associated with a major reduction in the level of consciousness, and the development of severe side effects such as excessive sedation, ataxia and disinhibition; their use should therefore be avoided in these situations (Sidtis *et al.*, 1993).

Dementia

Several lines of evidence support the efficacy of AZT in the treatment of HIV-associated dementia. The strongest evidence comes from a double-blind placebo-controlled study of patients with AIDS dementia complex (Sidtis *et al.*, 1993). In an earlier double-blind, placebo-controlled investigation, non-demented subjects with AIDS or AIDS-related complex (ARC) showed significant improvement in neuropsychological test performance while on AZT (Schmitt *et al.*, 1988). Supportive evidence is also available from a number of single-case studies and uncontrolled trials (Yarchoan *et al.*, 1987; Riccio *et al.*, 1990; Sanchez-Portocarrero *et al.*, 1996) and from natural experiments involving clinical cohorts (Portergies *et al.*, 1989). Although effective, the benefits of AZT are probably transient as they are apparent for a limited period of time. Nevertheless, given the fact that dementia tends to occur in advanced stages of HIV disease, a few months of improved quality of life is very significant.

Zidovudine may have a role in the prevention and treatment of HIV-associated dementia. Cohort studies have found better neuropsychological performance and better neuropsychological profile (Baldeweg *et al.*, 1995a,b) in people taking zidovudine, and neuropathological reports suggest that people treated with zidovudine (ZDV) have a lower incidence of multinucleated giant cells and HIV encephalitis (Gray *et al.*, 1994). A prospective double-blind placebo-controlled study of zidovudine in early HIV infection with a mean follow-up period of 28 months, found a significant increase in delta and theta slow frequency QEEG over the study period, and the slow wave amplitude remained unchanged in the zidovudine group, with no differences in neuropsychological function (Baldeweg *et al.*, 1995a,b).

The behavioural problems and mood disorders associated with HIV dementia can sometimes be treated with sedatives and major tranquillizers. Haloperidol has been recommended for the treatment of delirium, but there is a risk of serious side effects. The new atypical antipsychotics with selective dopamine D2 receptor blocking effect and absence of striatal action are a possible alternative, although their use should be carefully monitored. Stimulants have been advocated for people with low mood and cognitive impairment (Fernandez, Adams and Levy, 1988), but in view of the possible side effects (agitation, anorexia and elevated mood) and risk of misuse, they should be administered with caution.

Drug Misuse

In prescribing methadone to patients with HIV infection, several pharmacological interactions should be considered, particularly with anticonvulsants, antibiotics, antiviral medication and psychotropic drugs. Carbamazepine can diminish the plasmatic levels of methadone, triggering acute deprivation. The mechanism for this has yet to be clearly established, although it is well known that carbamazepine is an enzymatic inducer, and probably acts on the hepatic metabolism of methadone at the microsomal level. Therefore, in patients under methadone maintenance treatment who are also being treated with carbamazepine, it is necessary to increase the dosage of methadone and conduct plasmatic monitoring. These same considerations should be borne in mind when administering phenytoin.

An interaction has been described between rifampicin and methadone, since it enhances the hepatic metabolism of methadone, leading to early abstinence symptoms of opioid withdrawal. Patients who experience withdrawal while on methadone and rifampicin should be given increasing daily doses of methadone until withdrawal symptoms are prevented (Kreek *et al.*, 1976). Also, rifabutin can interfere with methadone, again making it necessary to increase the methadone dosage (Brown, Sawyer and Narang, 1996). Some patients on methadone maintenance exhibited a significant alteration in their handling of zidovudine, resulting in elevated levels of the antiviral agent (Schwartz *et al.*, 1992). Concerning psychotropic drugs, an increase in methadone plasma levels has been described after initiation of treatment with fluvoxamine (Bertschy *et al.*, 1994).

In a placebo-controlled study designed to assess the efficacy of fluoxetine treatment (40 mg/day) for cocaine dependency in HIV patients participating in a methadone treatment programme, the group of patients who received fluoxetine showed significantly lower levels of cocaine in their urine samples, as well as lower scores on craving evaluation scales. Fluoxetine was tolerated well, and judging from this study, it has a promising role in the treatment of cocaine abuse in this group (Batki *et al.*, 1993).

Pain

Pain is a common and debilitating symptom of HIV disease (Singer *et al.*, 1993) which is gravely underestimated and undertreated (Larue, Fontaine and Colleau, 1997), particularly among intravenous drug users, with AIDS (Breitbart *et al.*, 1995). One of the explanations for this phenomenon could be the fear of inducing or increasing drug addiction among these patients.

When managing pain in HIV disease, it is possible to apply the same principles as developed for cancer (World Health Organization, 1986). They involve the use of different psychotropic drugs (opioids, antidepressants, carbamazepine, psychostimulants), once the first-choice pain treatment drugs fail to control the symptoms.

Opiods

The use of opioids should depend on the intensity of pain, not the severity of prognosis. Clinicians frequently overestimate the duration of their effects. In hepatopathic patients, the dosage of opioids should be reduced, whereas in those with altered renal function the interval between doses should be increased. Special attention should be given to the possible development of pharmacological interactions between opiates and zidovudine. Morphine is metabolized by glucuronidation, just like the antiviral. If they are administered jointly, zidovudine may reach toxic levels (Miiller and Miller, 1988). To avoid this situation, caution is necessary when administering both agents, making the necessary dosage adjustments.

Tricyclic Antidepressants

Tricyclic antidepressants have been used in pain which fails to respond to opioids, as an adjuvant to analgesic drugs. They can be used in combination with regular analgesics in cases of neuropathic pain, with initial doses of 25–50mg at night (ONeill and Sherrard, 1993). Benefit should be apparent within 3–4 days. If not, the dose should be increased, up to 100mg/day. Antidepressant medication also has a heightening effect on the analgesia induced by morphine (France, Houpdt and Ellinwood, 1984), and can be used for this purpose in HIV-infected patients.

Low dosages of amitriptyline and nortriptyline have been recommended for the treatment of the chronic headaches that may appear in some patients with periseroconversion meningoencephalitis, and the painful symptoms of the predominantly sensory polyneuropathy associated with HIV-1 (Grant and Atkinson, 1996).

Carbamazepine

Carbamazepine is used in HIV-infected patients for its analgesic activity against the pain caused by peripheral nerve injury, whether due to direct viral infection or the development of treatment-related neurophathies. When it is being used, the haematopoietic function of these patients should be monitored closely, since they are frequently taking other medicaments, such as AZT, which can also cause toxic effects in bone marrow production.

Immunologic Effects of Psychotropic Drugs

A recent study by Leserman et al. (1997) showed that stress and depressive symptoms, especially when they occur jointly, are associated with decreased numbers of natural killer (NK) cells and CD8 + T lymphocytes in HIV-infected men, and they concluded there may be clinical implications for the cause of this disease. A different group evaluated immunologic effects of antidepressants in HIV positive patients and found no evidence of clinically significant adverse effects. They also found that HIV positive patients at all levels of immunosuppression tolerated the same doses, with the same frequency of side effects as medically healthy patients.

Psychotropics drugs have a wide variety of neuroendocrine and cellular effects which could affect immunologic function (Trzepacz, Dimartini and Tringali, 1993; Surman, 1993). Lithium has a proven effect on stimulation of the immunologic function and has been used as a therapeutic agent in a wide variety of chronic neutropenias (Barrett, 1980; Anderson, 1979). However, a favourable response to lithium depends on the integrity of the stem cell precursors. Lithium carbonate has been used in the treatment of zidovudine-associated neutropenia in AIDS patients without success (Worthington, 1990).

In vivo studies have shown opiates to promote HIV-1 replication in peripheral blood mononuclear cultures (Peterson *et al.*, 1990), while some studies in HIV negative individuals found that natural killer activity in parenteral heroin misusers was reduced compared to healthy controls or subjects on methadone maintenance (Brugo *et al.*, 1993; Novick *et al.*, 1989). There is no evidence that prescription of opiates to these patients has any impact on their immunity.

References

ANDERSON, T. (1979) 'Lithium carbonate stimulation of granulopoiesis in aemathologic and oncologic disease' *Arizona Medicine,* **36**, pp. 762–63.

AYUSO, J.L., BAYON, C., SANTO-DOMINGO, J. *et al.* (1989) 'Psychiatric aspects of patients with HIV infection in the general hospital', *Psychotherapy and Psychosomatics,* **52**, pp. 110–13.

AYUSO MATEOS, J.L., MONTAÑES, F., LASTRA, I. *et al.* (1997) 'HIV infection in psychiatric inpatients: an unlinked anonymous study', *British Journal of Psychiatry,* **170**, pp. 181–85.

BALDEWEG, T., CATALÁN, J., LOVETT, E. *et al.* (1995a) 'Long-term zidovudine neurocognitive deficits in HIV-1 infection', *AIDS,* **9**, pp. 589–96.

BALDEWEG, T., RICCIO, M., GRIZELIER, J. *et al.* (1995b) 'Neurophysiological evaluation of zidovudine in asymptomatic HIV-1 infection: a longitudinal placebo-controlled study', *Journal of Neurological Science,* **132**, pp. 162–69.

BARRET, A.J. (1980) 'Hematological effects of lithium and its use in treatment of neutropenia', *Blut,* **49**, pp. 1–6.

BATKI, S. (1990) 'Buspirone in drug users with AIDS or AIDS related complex', *Journal of Clinical Psychopharmacology,* **10**, pp. 111–15.

BERSTEIN, W.B. and SCHEROKMON, B. (1986) 'NMS in a patient with AIDS', *Acta Neurologica Scandinavia,* **73**, pp. 636–37.

BERTSCHY, G., BAUMANN, P., EAP, C.B. *et al.* (1994) 'Probable metabolic interaction between methadone and fluvoxamine in addict patients', *Drug Monitor,* **16**, pp. 42–45.

BREITBART,W., MAROTTA, R.F. and CALL, P. (1988) 'AIDS and neuroleptic malignant syndrome', *Lancet*, **2**, pp. 1488–89.

BREITBART, W.S., PASSIK, S., ROSENFELD, B. and McDONALD, M. (1995) 'Pain and psychological distress in substance abusers with AIDS: a comparison study of IDUs and non-IDUs', *Psychosomatics*, **36**, p. 175.

BREITBART, W., MAROTTA, R. *et al.* (1996) 'A double blind trial of haloperidol, chlorpromazine and lorazepam in the treatment of delirium in hospitalised AIDS patients', *American Journal of Psychiatry*, **153**, pp. 231–37.

BRODY, D., ADLER, L., KIM, T. *et al.* (1990) 'Effects of buspirone in seven schizophrenic subjects', *Journal of Clinical Psychopharmacology*, **10**, pp. 68–69.

BROWN, L.S., SAWYER, R.C. and NARANG, P.K. (1996) 'Evaluation of a possible pharmacologic interaction between rifabutin and methadone in HIV (+) injecting drug users', in Harris, L.S. (ed.) *Problems of drug dependence*, Rockville MD: DHHS Publications.

BURCH, E. and MONTOYA, J. (1989) 'NMS in an AIDS patient', *Journal of Clinical Psychopharmacology*, **9**, pp. 228–29.

CHIARELLO, R.J. and COLE, J.O. (1987) 'The use of psychostimulants in general psychiatry: a reconsideration', *Archives of General Psychiatry*, **44**, pp. 286–95.

DE SIMONE, C., CATANIA, S., TRINCHIERI, V. *et al.* (1988) 'Amelioration of the depression in HIV-infected subjects with L-acetyl carnitine therapy', *Journal of Drug Development*, **3**, pp. 163–66.

FERNANDEZ, F. and LEVY, J. (1990) 'Psychiatric diagnosis and pharmacotherapy of patients with HIV infection', *Review of Psychiatry*, Washington DC: American Psychiatric Press.

FERNANDEZ, F. and LEVY, J. (1991) 'Psychopharmacotherapy of psychiatric syndromes in asymptomatic and symptomatic HIV infection', *Psychiatric Medicine*, **9**, pp. 377–93.

FERNANDEZ, F. and LEVY, J. (1993) 'The use of molindone in the treatment of psychotic and delirious patients infected with the human immunodeficency virus', *General Hospital Psychiatry*, **15**, pp. 31–35.

FERNANDEZ, F., ADAMS, F. and LEVY, J.K. (1988) 'Cognitive impairment due to AIDS-related complex and its response to psychostimulants', *Psychosomatics*, **29**, pp. 38–46.

FRANCE, R.D., HOUPDT, J.L. and ELLINWOOD, E.H. (1984) 'Therapeutic effects of antidepresants in chronic pain', *General Hospital Psychiatry*, **6**, pp. 712–15.

GRANT, Y. and ATKINSON, J.H. (1996) 'Psychiatric aspects of acquired immune deficency syndrome', in Kaplan, H.I. and Sadock, B.J. (eds) *Textbook of Psychiatry*, New York: Williams & Wilkins, pp. 1644–69.

GRAY, F., BELEC, L., KEOHANE, C. *et al.* (1994) 'Zidovudine therapy and HIV encephalitis: a ten year neuropathological survey', *AIDS*, **8**, pp. 489–93.

HALMAN, M., WORTH, J.L., SANDERS, K. *et al.* (1993) 'Anticonvulsant use in the treatment of manic syndromes in patients with HIV1 infection', *Journal of Neuropsychiatry*, **54**, pp. 30–34.

HARRIS, M., JESTE, D. and GLEDHORN, A. (1991) 'New onset psychosis in HIV infected patients', *Journal of Clinical Psychiatry*, **52**, pp. 369–76.

HRISO, E., KUHN, T. and MASLEV, J. (1991) 'Extrapyramidal symptoms due to dopamine blocking agents in patients with AIDS encephalopathy', *American Journal of Psychiatry*, **148**, pp. 1558–61.

KAUFFMAN, M.W., CASSEM, N.H., MURRAY, G.B. *et al.* (1989) 'Use of psychostimulants in medically ill patients with neurological disease and major depression', *Canadian Journal of Psychiatry*, **29**, pp. 46–49.

KREEK, M.J., GARFIELD, J.W., GUTJAHR, C.L. and GIUISTI, L.M. (1976) 'Rifampin-induced methadone withdrawal', *New England Journal of Medicine*, **294**, pp. 1104–6.

LARUE, F., FONTAINE, A. and COLLEAU, S. (1997) 'Underestimation and undertreatment of pain in HIV disease: multicentric study', *British Medical Journal*, **314**, pp. 25–29.

LESERMAN, J., PETITTO, J.M., PERKINS, D.O., FOLDS, J.D., GOLDEN, R.N. and EVANS, D.L. (1997) 'Severe stess, depressive symptoms and changes in lymphocyte subset in human immunodeficiency virus-infected men', *Archives of General Psychiatry*, **54**, pp. 279–85.

LIPINSKI, J.F., MALLYA, G., ZIMMERMAN, P. *et al.* (1989) 'Fluoxetine induced akathisia: clinical and theoretical implications', *Journal Clinical Psychiatry*, **50**, pp. 339–42.

MANNING, D., JACOBSBERG, L., ERHART, S., PERRY, S. and FRANCES, A. (1990) 'The efficacy of imipramine in the treatment of HIV related depression' paper, presented at the International Conference on AIDS, San Francisco.

MILLER, L.G. and MILLER, M. (1988) 'Drug selection for rheumatic manifestations of aquired immunodeficiency syndrome', *American Journal of Medicine*, **85**, pp. 894–95.

NATH, A., JANCKOVIC, J. and PATTIGREW, L.C. (1987) 'Movement disorders and AIDS', *Neurology*, **37**, pp. 37–41.

OCHITILL, H. (1992) 'Prescribing psychotropic drugs for patients with AIDS', *Drug Therapy*, **22**, pp. 37–42.

O'NEILL, W.M. and SHERRARD, J.S. (1993) 'Pain in human immunodeficiency virus disease: a review', *Pain*, **54**, pp. 3–14.

OSTROW, D., GRANT, I. and ATKINSON, H. (1988) 'Assesment and management of the AIDS patient with neuropsychiatric disturbances', *Journal of Clinical Psychiatry*, **49**, pp. 14–22.

PERETTA, P., NISITA, C., ZACCAGNINI, E. *et al.* (1992) 'Effect of Bromperidol on HIV related psychosis in a sample of seropositive patients with brain damage', paper presented at the International Conference on AIDS, Amsterdam (abstracts VIII).

PETERSON, P.K., SHARP, B., SEKKERT, G. *et al.* (1990) Morphine promotes the growth of HIV in human peripheral mononuclear cell cocultives', *Journal of Acquired Immune Deficiency Syndrome,* **4**, pp. 869–73.

PORTERGIES, P., DE GANS, J., LANGE, J.M.A. *et al.* (1989) 'Declining evidence of AIDS dementia complex after introduction of zidovudine treatment', *British Medical Journal,* **299**, pp. 818–21.

RABKIN, J.G. and HARRISON, W.M. (1990) 'Effect of imipramine on depression and immune status in a sample of men with HIV infection', *American Journal of Psychiatry* **147**, pp. 495–97.

RABKIN, R. and RABKIN, J.G. (1995) 'Testosterone effects on mood in late-stage HIV illness', *Psychosomatics,* **36**, p. 175.

RABKIN, J.G., RABKIN, R. and WAGNER, G. (1994) 'Effects of fluoxetine on mood and immune status in depressed patients with HIV illness', *Journal of Clinical Psychiatry,* **155**, pp. 92–97.

RABKIN, J.G., WAGNER, G. and RABKIN, R. (1994) 'Effects of sertraline on mood and immune status in patients with major depression and HIV illness: open trial', *Journal of Clinical Psychiatry,* **55**, pp. 433–39.

RABKIN, J.G., RABKIN, R., HARRISON, W. and WAGNER, G. (1994) 'Imipramine effects on mood in depressed patients with HIV illness', *American Journal of Psychiatry,* **151**, pp. 516–23.

RICCIO, M., BURGESS, A., HAWKINS, D. *et al.* (1990) 'Neuropsychological and psychiatric changes following treatment of ARC patients with zidovudine', *International Journal of STD and AIDS,* **1**, pp. 435–37.

SANCHEZ-PORTOCARRERO, J., JIMENEZ-ESCRIG, A., PEREZ-CECILIA, E., AYUSO MATEOS, J.L., ROCA, V., RUIZ-YAGUE, M., BARQUERO, M., RAMIREZ, C. and VARELA, E. (1996) 'AIDS dementia complex: incidence, clinical profile and impact of zidovudine treatment', *European Journal of Neurology,* **3**, pp. 191–97.

SCHMITT, F.A., BIGLEY, J.W., MCKINNIS, R., LOGUE, P.E., EVANS, R.W. and DRUCKER, J.L. (1988) 'Neuropsychological outcome of zidovudine treatment of patients with AIDS and ARC', *New England Journal of Medicine,* **319**, pp. 1573–78.

SCHWARTZ, E.L., BRECHBÜHL, A.-B., KAHL, P. *et al.* (1992) 'Pharmacokinetic interactions of zidovudine and methadone in intravenous drug-using patients with HIV infection', *Journal of Aquired Immune Deficiency Syndrome,* **5**, pp. 619–26.

SCURLOCK, H., SINGH, A.N. and CATALÁN, J. (1995) 'Atypical antipsychotic drugs in the treatment of manic syndromes in patients with HIV1 infection', *Journal of Psychopharmacology,* **9**, pp. 151–54.

SHEDLACK, K.J., SOLDATO-COUTURE, C.S. and SWANSON, C.L. (1994) 'Rapidly progressive tardive dyskinesia in AIDS', *Biological Psychiatry,* **35**, pp. 147–48.

SIDTIS, J.J., GATSONIS, C., PRICE, R.W. *et al.* (1993) 'Zidovudine treatment of AIDS dementia complex: placebo-controlled trial', *Annals of Neurology,* **33**, pp. 342–49.

SINGER, E.J., ZORILLA, C., FAHY-CHANDON, B. *et al.* (1993) 'Painful symptoms reported by ambulatory HIV-infected men in a longitudinal study', *Pain*, **54**, pp. 15–19.

SINGH, A. and CATALÁN, J. (1994) 'Risperidone in HIV-related manic psychosis', *Lancet*, **344**, pp. 1029–30.

SINGH, A. and CATALÁN, J. (1996) 'The efficacy of selective serotonin reuptake inhibitors (SSRIs) for the treatment of depression in patients with symptomatic HIV infection', *Journal of Serotonin Research*, **4**, pp. 237–41.

SINGH, A., GALLEDGE, H. and CATALÁN, J. (1997) 'Treatment of HIV related psychotic disorders with risperidone: a series of 21 cases', *Journal of Psychosomatic Research*, **42**, 5, pp. 113–16.

SINGH, A., SCURLOCK, H. and CATALÁN, J. (1995) 'Paroxetine induced erectile dysfunction succesfully treated with yohimbine in patients suffering from HIV infection', *Journal of Serotonin Research*, **4**, pp. 283–85.

STEFAN, M. and CATALÁN, J. (1995) 'Psychiatric patients and HIV infection: a new population at risk', *British Journal of Psychiatry*, **167**, pp. 721–27.

SURMAN, O.S. (1993) 'Possible immunological effects of psychotropic medication', *Psychosomatics*, **35**, pp. 139–43.

TRACHMAN, S.B. (1992) 'Buspirone-induced psychosis in a human immunodeficency virus-infected man', *Psychosomatics*, **33**, pp. 332–35.

TRZEPACZ, P., DIMARTINI, A. and TRINGALI, R. (1993) Psychopharmacological issues in organ transplantation. Part 2: psychopharmacological medications', *Psychosomatics*, **34**, pp. 290–98.

WAGNER, G.J., RABKIN, J.G. and RABKIN, R. (1997) 'Dextroamphetamine as a treatment for depression and low energy in AIDS patients: a pilot study', *Journal of Psychosomatic Research*, **42**, pp. 407–11.

WOLCOTT, D.L., FAWZY, F.I. and PASNAU, R.O. (1985) 'AIDS and consultation-liaison psychiatry', *General Hospital Psychiatry*, **7**, pp. 280–92.

WORLD HEALTH ORGANIZATION (1986) *Cancer Pain Relief*. Geneva: WHO.

WORLD HEALTH ORGANIZATION (1990) *Report on the second consultation on the neuropsychiatric aspects of HIV-1 infection*, Geneva: WHO Global Programme on AIDS.

WORTHINGTON, M. (1990) 'Lack of effect of lithium carbonate on zidovudine-associated neutropenia in patients with AIDS', *Journal of Infectious Diseases*, **162**, pp. 777–78.

YARCHOAN, R., BERG, G., BOUWERS, P. *et al.* (1987) 'Response of HIV-associated neurological disease to zidovudine', *Lancet*, **i**, pp. 132–35.

Chapter 10

Cognitive-Behavioural Therapy and HIV Risk Sexual Behaviour

Susan Thornton and Deepti Shah

This chapter focuses on face-to-face interventions for prevention of HIV trans-mission, particularly cognitive-behavioural approaches to sexual behaviour change. No attempt has been made to carry out an exhaustive review since several are already available (Kelly, 1995; Oakley, Fullerton and Holland, 1995; Kalichman, Carey and Johnson, 1997a). Instead, the aim is to highlight the complex psychological problems faced by some individuals among which sexual risk behaviour is only one of many interlinked problems. In providing a service aimed at helping HIV/genitourinary medicine clinic attenders to adopt and maintain safer sex, it has been apparent there are many obstacles to behaviour change, and perhaps myths about what constitutes an appropriate strategy in the late 1990s. The lessons learned from this service form the core of what follows.

Introduction

It is estimated that by the year 2000 more than 40 million people worldwide will be infected with HIV and currently 16,000 people a day are newly diag-nosed. Since the start of the epidemic, almost 12 million people have died (UNAIDS/WHO, 1997). By far the most common transmission route is sexual contact, and one in every 100 adults in the sexually active age group 15–49 was living with HIV infection in 1997. A vaccine is still a remote hope for the future, and while the new antiretroviral treatments have improved the lives of many to whom they have been available, they do not constitute a cure. Preven-tion of HIV risk sexual behaviour remains a priority for the foreseeable future. It is well known that the overwhelming majority of HIV-infected people live in the developing world, and major changes in political, socio-economic and organizational policies will be necessary to stem the epidemic. It is therefore critically important that firstly, a global strategy for behavioural science based efforts towards prevention is implemented, and secondly, that the developed countries maintain funding to multilateral initiatives and research in the areas which have been devastated by AIDS and those in which the spread of HIV infection is increasing (Coates *et al.*, 1996).

The stark figures quoted above are daunting indeed, but after more than fifteen years of the epidemic, how well have we, in the developed countries, coped with preventing people from becoming infected with HIV? All the advantages of well-developed communications, well-financed health care and research, together with relatively high standards of living, have been available to those in most Western countries, and vast sums of money have been poured into health promotion and prevention initiatives. For example, in 1997/98 the amount spent on gay men's HIV prevention services in inner London in the voluntary sector alone, amounted to well over £1.5 million. Although there has been a drop in the numbers of infections in many European countries and the United States, incidence of new infections remains unacceptably high among some groups of the population and in some geographical areas. In particular, there is evidence that younger people are most at risk. The prevalence of HIV seropositivity among young gay men in San Francisco is only marginally below the figure for 1984, at a time when the threat of AIDS was not yet recognized (Osmond *et al.*, 1994). Half of all new infections in the United States occur in people younger than 25 years (Rosenberg, 1994).

Prevention Strategies

Strategies for the prevention of HIV infection range from the dissemination of information to the provision of clean blood supplies. As has been shown in very many studies, being well informed about HIV transmission is not by itself sufficient to prevent risk behaviour. It is, however, necessary to ensure that young people are not denied the knowledge they need to protect themselves. There is unequivocal evidence that early sex education does not increase promiscuity among young people (Wellings *et al.*, 1995) and can decrease high risk sexual activity (Kirby *et al.*, 1991), but there is still some resistance to education about sex and prevention of sexually transmitted disease (STD) in schools. The effectiveness of needle exchange programmes for injecting drug users in reducing HIV transmission is also now well established (Hurley, Jolley and Kaldor, 1997).

Changing sexual behaviours has proved more difficult. Unfortunately, while HIV test counselling is clearly important in helping people to make appropriate decisions, there is no evidence that it has any impact on sexual risk behaviour among those testing negative (Zenilman *et al.*, 1992; Otten *et al.*, 1993). The concept of 'negotiated safety' has been advanced (Kippax *et al.*, 1993), in which apparently risky sex among gay men is in fact a negotiated agreement to have unprotected intercourse between partners who identify themselves as having the same serostatus, hence making it a low risk activity. Stall and Ekstrand (1994) accept that variables identified in quantitative research are not sufficient to explain interpersonal and contextual issues in sexual risk behaviour and endorse the need for qualitative data to help in constructing theories to explain maintenance or otherwise of safer sex. They insist, however, that if qualitative analyses proceed without reference to the one quantitative variable whose validity is not contestable, namely high rates of seroconversion among gay men, they will not be addressing the critical issue.

Findings in two qualitative studies have suggested that negotiated safety accounts for little of the occurrence of unprotected intercourse. Ridge (1996) has pointed out that some of the prerequisites for negotiated safety which include open verbal communication and an equal balance of power were not common in his small study of gay relationships. In another qualitative study (Sharp *et al.*, 1996) the authors report that almost half the men in their sample of 35 deviated from the conditions necessary for negotiated safety and engaged in unsafe activity. In addition, evidence exists that while those who report frequent engagement in unsafe sex may make a positive choice to do so, perhaps in the context of a stable relationship, many men who have occasional high risk episodes report negative emotional consequences, including guilt, worry, fear and discouragement, suggesting their behaviour was not the rational choice implied by the idea of negotiated safety (Ekstrand *et al.*, 1992).

Designing interventions for sexual risk behaviour which work and finding appropriate methods to assess their effectiveness has not been easy. In a critical review of 68 evaluations of interventions aimed at changing HIV risk behaviours, Oakley, Fullerton and Holland (1995) judged that almost three-quarters failed to meet adequate methodological criteria. Among the 18 studies judged to be methodologically sound, only five interventions were effective. Two were course-based and increased AIDS knowledge (Di Clemente *et al.*, 1989; Walter and Vaughan, 1993) as well as positive changes in beliefs, self-efficacy and risk behaviours (Walter and Vaughan, 1993) among high school students. Three were skills-based programmes which were effective in reducing favourable attitudes to risky sex and intentions to engage in it among Black adolescent males (Jemmott, Jemmott and Fong, 1992) and both decreased risk behaviours and increased consistent condom use among homeless adolescents (Rotheram-Borus *et al.*, 1991). The remaining intervention was a 12-week group intervention for gay men which reduced reported frequency of unprotected intercourse to near zero levels and increased condom use, changes which were largely maintained at 16-month follow-up (Kelly *et al.*, 1989). The authors of the review conclude that sound and effective interventions are likely to be skills-based and delivered by peers or clinical psychologists.

A more recent review (Kalichman, Carey and Johnson, 1997) specifically addressed controlled studies of interventions which aimed at changing sexual risk behaviour and were grounded in the principles of social learning theory. Features which were central to all the interventions were education about and sensitization to risk, building of self-efficacy through skills training, including communication, negotiation, condom use, behavioural self-management and problem-solving skills. These are also key elements in a cognitive-behavioural approach. Meta-analytic statistical techniques were used to determine the effect sizes of the twelve selected interventions. This is essentially a measure of change in the intervention group participants compared with those in the control group on the risk outcome measures used in each study. All the effect sizes were positive ranging from .11 for a single-session intervention for gay men to .53 for a six-session programme for adolescents. All the studies involved group interventions and most were published in the 1990s.

Cognitive-Behavioural Interventions for Individuals

In the United Kingdom, the largest proportion of HIV infections and AIDS cases have consistently been reported from the London area. The great majority of these are among gay men and there is evidence of a continuing high incidence among this group in London (Evans *et al.*, 1993; Miller *et al.*, 1995). The number of gay men diagnosed with HIV in 1996 was the highest of any year since recording began and in 1997, numbers were very close to those recorded ten years ago (Communicable Disease Report, 1998). A recent survey of sexual lifestyles among 1,200 gay men found that at least three-quarters of the respondents had casual sexual encounters and that one in three sexual acts was unsafe (Project Zorro, reported in the *Independent*, 30 March, 1998). There is also evidence that substantial numbers of HIV positive individuals are attending for treatment of new STDs (Catchpole *et al.*, 1996), and others known to the clinics and with a history of previous negative HIV tests are returning to test positive (Gray *et al.*, 1997).

A large number of studies have sought to identify correlates and predictors of HIV sexual risk behaviour among gay men. Methodological and sample diversity and the fact that sexual behaviour is subject to individual, social and cultural influences results in findings which are at times inconclusive or contradictory. For example, the operational definition of what constitutes risk behaviour may be in terms of frequency of unprotected intercourse, proportion of unprotected episodes, number of partners, number of partners of unknown HIV serostatus, or some combination of these. The timing of the study and its geographical location in relation to prevalence and awareness of the infection may also affect the findings. Increasingly, it seems prudent to assess the factors relevant to risk behaviour in the specific population being targeted and design an intervention which addresses these factors, rather than relying on research findings which are often too broad in their quality.

In 1993 members of our unit established a sexual risk reduction service for HIV/genitourinary medicine (GUM) clinic attenders in central London, offering cognitive behavioural intervention by clinical psychologists. The HIV/GUM clinics served more than 2000 HIV-infected people, over 80 per cent of whom are gay men. While outcome data suggests that direct face-to-face contact is most effective in changing sexual risk behaviour (Choi and Coates, 1994; Kalichman, Carey and Johnson, 1997), it is well known that getting people to attend face-to-face interventions for risk reduction is problematic (McKirnan, Ostrow and Hope, 1996) and attendance at the risk reduction service has been no exception. Although clinic staff are aware of many individuals who are engaging in risk behaviour, few attenders acknowledge this or agree to contact either the health advisors or the risk reduction service. Referrals have remained relatively constant at between 50 and 70 per 12-month period but one-third of those referred fail to attend their first appointment and almost one-fifth of those who do attend drop out of the intervention. To date, the ages of those referred range from 18 to 72 and the great majority (83 per cent) were gay men, about one-fifth of whom were HIV positive.

Based on the available research, it was originally expected to provide cognitive-behavioural groups modelled on the successful intervention of Kelly *et al.* (1989). This group intervention included HIV risk education, cognitive-behavioural self-management and assertiveness skills training, together with problem solving related to lifestyle and establishing social supports. We found, however, that there were high rates of psychiatric and psychological disorder among those referred, and the presenting problems were so heterogeneous that a group approach was not possible. Among the first 50 individuals assessed for intervention, more than half (57 per cent) had a past history of treatment for psychological or psychiatric disorders (Thornton *et al.*, 1994). More recent data shows that psychiatric morbidity as assessed by the GHQ-28 (Goldberg and Hillier, 1979) is high. Currently, more than three-quarters of attenders score within the range denoting a psychiatric case. At least half are also problem drinkers, as defined by scores on the CAGE questionnaire (Mayfield, McLeod and Hall, 1974) and many make regular use of recreational drugs.

Standard measures of psychological morbidity did not seem to capture the mixed symptomatology and difficulties seen in many of the risk reduction attenders, and 52 individuals who were consecutive referrals attending for their first appointment were asked to complete the MMPI-2 (Hathaway and McKinley, 1989). This inventory is one of the most widely used tests of personality and is considered to be useful clinically for distinguishing between adjustment and abnormality (Helmes and Reddon, 1993). Average scores were abnormally high for 5 of the 10 clinical scales and the F scale, which forms part of the validity scales and is an indicator of overall psychopathology (Meyer, 1993), was also raised above the cut-off level. Two-thirds of the sample had abnormally high average scores (Scragg, Shah and Thornton, in press). This finding provides convergent validity for the clinical observation of severe and long-standing psychopathology as well as personality problems among many of the risk reduction attenders.

The MMPI-2 is a very long questionnaire, unsuitable for routine use, and the EPQ-R (Eysenck and Eysenck, 1991) is now used as a pre-intervention measure of personality. It has 90 items in the form of simple statements to be endorsed yes or no. It measures the personality dimensions of extraversion, neuroticism and psychoticism. This questionnaire has highly satisfactory reliability and the validity of its scales is the best supported of any personality measure (Kline, 1993). Average scores on the neuroticism and psychoticism dimensions are high and well above the normal range. Individuals who score high on neuroticism tend to be anxious, to worry, be moody and frequently depressed, whereas high scorers on psychoticism tend to be tough-minded, disregarding of social rules, lacking in empathy, hostile and solitary with difficulty in fitting into society.

A relatively high proportion of participants (23 per cent) report unwanted sexual experiences in childhood, which reflects recent evidence of a strong association between unsafe sexual behaviour among gay men and childhood sexual abuse (Strathdee *et al.*, 1996; Jinich *et al.*, 1998). There is evidence that sexual abuse in childhood among males may have a wide range of effects, including depression, poor self-concept, difficulty in establishing and maintaining relationships, sexual dysfunction and sexual compulsion (Cahill, Llewellyn and Pearson, 1991). All of this documents what is found clinically: many of those who are having difficulties with safer sex have complex problems sometimes rooted in a difficult childhood which has contributed to unhelpful personality traits and maladaptive coping. Of course, not all the participants have these difficulties; but when they are present, a straightforward intervention addressing only risk reduction is rarely appropriate.

Personality and Unsafe Sex

The possibility of links between personality factors or problems and sexual risk behaviour is only recently beginning to be addressed, and a number of articles have appeared in the last two years which look at the contribution of what may broadly be described as personality factors to unsafe sex. In a report from a longitudinal study, sexual adventurism assessed using a scale based on a measure of sexual sensation seeking (Kalichman *et al.*, 1994) was an important predictor of HIV infection. Almost 80 per cent of those seroconverting in the nine-year period under review scored above the median on sexual adventurism (Di Franceisco, Ostrow and Chmiel, 1996). Another study showed that sexual impulsivity was a significant predictor of unprotected intercourse among both HIV positive and HIV negative men (Hays *et al.*, 1997).

Kalichman *et al.* (1997) assessed fatalistic thinking and life satisfaction using standardized measures together with perceived life expectancy among 430 gay men and examined the relationship of these variables to risk behaviour. Men who engaged in unprotected anal intercourse outside exclusive relationships had higher fatalism and lower life satisfaction scores as well as shorter perceived life expectation than men who practised only safer sex and those in exclusive relationships. The results of this study suggest that risky sexual behaviour may be associated with unhappiness and a lack of hope for the future, at least for some.

In a study carried out in our local HIV/GUM clinics, 175 attenders completed the NEO five-factor personality inventory (Costa and McRae, 1992) and a short questionnaire assessing self-reported unsafe sexual behaviour.

There was an association of risk behaviour with low agreeableness among heterosexuals and with low conscientiousness among gay men (Scragg, 1995). Two studies have looked at the association between personality disorders and HIV serostatus. A higher prevalence of personality disorders was found among gay HIV-infected men than among those who were negative (Perkins *et al.*, 1994); and in a study of hospital inpatients (Ellis, Collis and King, 1994), borderline personality disorder was diagnosed more frequently among HIV positive patients than among control patients.

Personality disorder was also found to be a significant predictor of sexual risk-taking behaviour among GUM clinic attenders in London (Ellis, Collis and King, 1995). These findings concur with what has been seen in our risk reduction service, in suggesting that intervention to promote safer sex behaviours may be complicated by personality factors.

Cognitive-Behavioural Model

A cognitive-behavioural model of risky sexual behaviour (Figure 10.1) has been developed from our experience (Tallis, 1995) and, in particular, informed by the work of Gold (Gold *et al.*, 1991; Gold and Skinner, 1992; Gold, Skinner and Ross, 1994; Gold and Rosenthal, 1995), who has drawn attention to the powerful effect of cognitive processes, in the form of self-justifications, on unsafe sexual behaviour. The model of risky sexual behaviour is based on the work of Beck, first described more than twenty years ago (Beck, 1976) and elaborated in many publications since then. The cognitive model is about understanding the links between cognition, emotion, physical feelings and behaviour. Cognition may be in the form of events (thoughts, memories, images), structures (assumptions, attitudes, beliefs) or processes (biases in thinking). A person's beliefs, thoughts and interpretation of events, rather than the events themselves, may trigger emotional, physiological and behavioural responses, and they also play a powerful role in maintaining dysfunctional moods and behaviours. Strong emotions tend to generate more extreme thinking and a narrowing in the focus of attention. Three levels of cognition are relevant:

Automatic Thoughts

Automatic thoughts are the moment-to-moment, unplanned thoughts (words, images, memories) that flow through one's mind throughout the day. People may not be immediately aware of them but they are accessible, e.g. I can't stand it; nothing I do works; I think I'm going to enjoy this. The important point about them is that they are accepted without question as if they are facts and they influence one's mood and behaviour. Automatic thoughts are linked to assumptions.

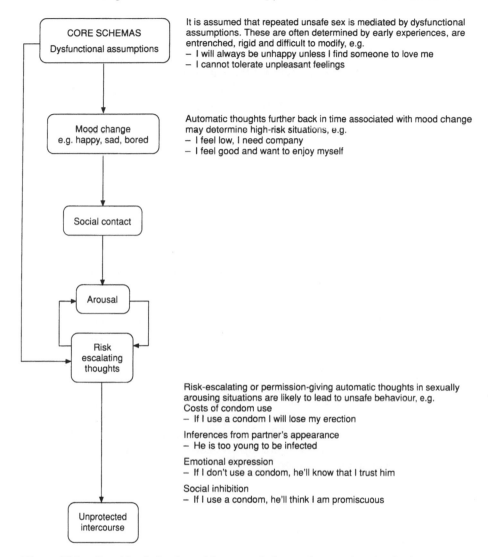

Figure 10.1 *Cognitive-behavioural framework for working with individuals.*

Assumptions

Assumptions are the beliefs or rules which guide our behaviour and expectations, and they often drive our automatic thinking. They include 'should', 'must' and 'ought' beliefs, e.g. a person should always think of others first; I must stay in control. They include 'if...then' beliefs, e.g. if I get close to anyone, they will reject me; if I don't find someone to love me, I will never be happy. These underlying assumptions are rarely articulated consciously.

Schemas

Schemas are absolute, rigid, self-perpetuating (and therefore resistant to change) core beliefs about oneself, others and the world, e.g. I am helpless; I must have someone to lean on; I am unlovable; I am special; people will hurt, cheat, take advantage. As with dysfunctional assumptions, they are seldom easily accessible. Schemas are assumed to develop during childhood when they are probably reasonable, valid ways of the child making sense of the environment he or she happens to be in. They are elaborated over time until they are so familiar that they are unquestioned, as are the assumptions and automatic thoughts which are linked to them.

Biases and Distortions

Automatic thoughts are subject to biases and distortions, which means they do not fit all the facts and they prevent one from attending to the meaning of all the available information. Some of the most common are black and white or dichotomous thinking (people are either good or bad; I never attract anyone; nobody likes me); jumping to conclusions on the basis of one event (he didn't look, he can't stand me; he is too young to be infected); arbitrary inference (if he uses a condom, he must be positive; if he uses a condom, he must be negative). The process of therapy encourages clients to view their thoughts as hypotheses or guesses, not facts, and to generate alternatives. This is achieved in a collaborative manner in which therapist and client together explore the possibilities and test them out. The basis of cognitive behavioural therapy is that behaviour and patterns of thinking are learned and new ways of behaving and thinking can also be learned.

Using the Model

The model in Figure 10.1 provides a framework within which to identify the appropriate way of working with a particular individual. For some, the intervention focuses on the risk-escalating or permission-giving automatic thoughts which occur in the sexual situation and which tend to become more accessible with sexual arousal. For others, it may be necessary to work at the level of dysfunctional assumptions or core schemas (Young, 1990; Padesky, 1994). Behavioural techniques are an integral part of the approach as well as the teaching of behavioural skills. Many individuals have social anxieties, assertiveness deficits and performance anxiety in sexual situations. Graded exposure, role play, condom practice and behavioural experiments are often useful. Some patients lack the basic condom skills necessary for their effective use and a condom demonstrator is routinely used to assess this.

Since cognitive events and processes are often the focus of intervention, it was necessary to develop an instrument to assess risk-escalating thoughts and any changes following intervention. The sexual risk cognitions questionnaire (SRCQ) is a 22-item instrument with additional 8–12 item subsections designed for groups defined by gender, sexual orientation and HIV serostatus (Shah, Thornton and Burgess, 1997). The items are rated on a five-point scale from 'never had thought' to 'very frequently had thought'. Some examples are given below:

- I'm sure he's HIV negative. I can just tell.
- I want to show him he is somebody special.
- My positive state of mind can prevent me from being infected.
- If he chooses not to use a condom, he must be infected as well.
- We've both had HIV positive tests, so there's nothing to lose for either of us.
- It's his responsibility to use a condom: I'm not responsible for others.

In addition to the measures of personality and psychological morbidity described above, risk reduction attenders also complete self-report measures assessing sexual risk behaviour, problem drinking, social anxiety and confidence in the ability to maintain safer sex rated on a seven-point scale from 'not at all confident' to 'completely confident'. Two case studies are presented to illustrate the approach. Personal details have been changed to protect the identities of the people concerned.

KC is a Gay Man, Age 21

This man's sexual risk behaviour was maintained by his cognitions and by lack of condom skills as well as by enjoyment of unprotected sex. In this case, although he had relatively high scores on the GHQ-28 and used recreational drugs and alcohol, there were no severe current psychological problems or history of psychiatric illness.

Assessment

Similar to its application in other problem areas, the aim of cognitive-behavioural assessment is to agree a formulation of the sexual risk behaviour with the person, and gather detailed information about factors maintaining the behaviour. The individual is educated about the cognitive-behavioural model and the risk behaviour is analyzed in terms of antecedent behaviours and beliefs and their consequences. The relationship of triggers, both external and internal, and automatic thoughts to unsafe behaviour is identified. Automatic thoughts are evoked in sexually arousing situations and may directly impair impulse control.

KC had his first sexual encounter with a man at the age of 15 years. At this time, he was very aware of the possible risk of HIV infection and of the importance of safer sex. In fact, he practised safer sex only for the next five years. He was always the passive partner during anal intercourse. Eighteen months earlier, however, he had engaged in unprotected passive and active anal intercourse with a casual partner. He was not sure why he was unsafe, but remembers being encouraged by his sexual partner. He felt that the sex was 'amazing' and recalled that the 'risk was the thrill'. At the time he was referred, he was regularly having unsafe sex: on the 20 occasions he had had intercourse in the previous three months, 8 contacts were unprotected. He never used a condom if he was the active partner, and he never initiated the use of a condom by his partners. He believed that if his sexual partners were young and attractive, they were less likely to be HIV positive. He also believed his partners if they said they were not positive. He had an HIV test soon after his first unsafe sexual encounter. The test was negative and this reinforced KC's confidence in his ability to judge a person's HIV status based on their appearance and personality. He had not had an HIV test since.

KC often took ecstasy and alcohol before or during sex and was more likely to be unsafe with drugs or alcohol, although he acknowledged he was also unsafe when completely sober. He stated, 'If I was positive, I would be completely safe,' and he believed that other people would follow the same rule. It also became clear that KC lost his erection if he used or contemplated using a condom.

Treatment

Over a three-month period, KC was seen on eight occasions. The precipitants for the risk behaviour were identified in a number of ways, including free recall of a recent unsafe sexual encounter, responses in the SRCQ, thought records and the sexual diary which KC kept throughout the treatment (Figure 10.2). He was taught techniques to challenge risk-escalating thoughts by self-questioning and developing accurate appraisals of risk. He was asked to demonstrate condom use with a plastic condom demonstrator, in order to assess whether he had the behavioural skills necessary for efficient condom use. This is also a useful method for eliciting any negative thoughts and feelings about condoms.

THERAPIST (TH): What is going through your mind as you are opening the packet of condoms?

KC: It will ruin the sex.

TH: How?

KC: It won't feel as sensual.

TH: Have there been times when a condom has been used and it has felt sensual?

Time	Type of sexual contact					Type of partner			Where did you have sex?					Substances?		General mood? e.g. Depressed anxious
	Anal, were you:		Oral, were you:		Were condoms used	Regular	casual	other	cruis-ing	Cottag-ing	club	own home	partner's home	alcohol	drugs	
	active	passive	being suck-ed	suck-ing												

Please make a note for every sexual contact you have – tick the appropriate columns

Figure 10.2 *Sexual behaviour diary.*

KC:	Yes.
TH:	What was different then?
KC:	I was passive, I didn't have to put the condom on.
TH:	What's so bad about wearing a condom?
KC:	I will lose my erection.

Since for KC the perceived costs of using a condom outweighed the benefits, the advantages and disadvantages of using a condom were elicited in order to help him appraise his view more explicitly. He identified the following advantages and disadvantages.

Advantages	Disadvantages
Clean	Lack of intimacy
Feel better about self afterwards	No skin-to-skin contact
Taking responsibility	Breaks flow of sex
	Excitement of taking risk

The disadvantages were challenged and the advantages highlighted.

TH: How much better is sex without a condom? How much better on a scale of one to a hundred per cent?
KC: Ten to thirty per cent.
TH: Are there any ways of improving sex with a condom?
KC: Don't know.
TH: For example, one can focus on sensations of other parts of the body. Can you think of other ways?
KC: Being relaxed.
TH: Using fantasies?

Continuum methods (Padesky, 1994) were used to challenge dichotomous thinking (e.g. sex is only good without a condom). This approach helps to shift absolutist beliefs to more balanced mid-range positions. KC was also taught to replace risk-escalating thoughts about the consequences of condom use with risk-reducing thoughts. These risk-reducing thoughts ranged from simple statements such as 'I must use a condom' to questions such as 'Is it worth the risk?'.

Since one of KC's main anxieties about his own condom use was that he would lose his erection, he was asked to use graded behavioural exercises at home, including masturbation with a condom using the stop-start technique. The aim of this was to teach KC that he could maintain an erection with a condom. He underestimated the likelihood of his contracting HIV infection and also stated that he was willing to take this risk. KC's perception of his personal risk of contracting HIV was challenged using a number of techniques. For example, he was asked to form an accurate appraisal of personal risk in percentage terms.

TH: What is the chance of you becoming HIV positive?
KC: Twenty per cent chance of becoming HIV positive. I'm willing to take that risk.
TH: Are there other situations in which there is a twenty per cent chance of something dangerous happening to you?
KC: Swimming in the sea with sharks, twenty per cent chance of being bitten.
TH: Are you willing to take this risk?
KC: Never.

His belief in his ability to judge a person's HIV status based on their appearance was also challenged. KC estimated that there was a small (20 per cent) chance of his partner being positive if he had any of these attributes:

• He works full time in a 'respectable' job, e.g. solicitor.
• He looks fit.
• He seems intelligent and sensible.
• He does not seem promiscuous.
• He is young.

The thinking errors *jumping to conclusions* and *overgeneralization* were identified. KC minimized the fact that he was willing to be unsafe and maximized the importance of a partner's characteristics. The prejudice model (Padesky, 1995) was discussed with him to highlight the thinking errors he made to facilitate unsafe sex. This model is one in which the individual is shown that a belief can be seen in the same light as a prejudice, and that information which supports the belief is quickly incorporated while information which does not is discounted or ignored, just as with a prejudice. Finally, KC had difficulty in asserting his own needs and effectively communicating the safer-sex message to his partners. Various cognitive-behavioural strategies were used to enhance his skills in these areas.

Outcome

After three months of therapy, KC had learned to successfully challenge his negative cognitions regarding condoms and had learned to use them without fear of losing his erection. He rated himself as more confident about maintaining safer sex and he was no longer taking alcohol or drugs to have sex. Before intervention he reported that 40 per cent, of his penetrative sex encounters were unprotected, and at the end of treatment this had dropped to zero. At 3-month follow-up he reported only two unprotected encounters, which represented 6 per cent of penetrative sex occasions; and at 6-month follow-up he reported only one. His scores in the GHQ-28 and the SRCQ dropped from 14 and 83 respectively at pretreatment to 5 and 46 at 6-month follow-up.

FD is a Gay Man, Age 26

This case highlights the importance of core schemas in maintaining risk behaviour. FD was born and brought up in rural Spain and had come to the United Kingdom five years previously to work as a head waiter. His reasons for leaving Spain were that he felt he would have greater job opportunities in the United Kingdom and because he had to lead a false life in Spain. His elderly parents, five older siblings and most of his friends knew nothing of his sexual orientation.

Assessment

FD presented with low mood and anxiety, including panic attacks. He reported that he often felt people were looking at him or talking behind his back, and this frequently led him to avoid going out. He also avoided public transport and crowded places for the same reasons. He described a vicious cycle of negative ruminations and social withdrawal. He reported that when he was feeling like this, he sometimes forced himself to go out to meet friends but inevitably would drink too much and become verbally aggressive, accusing others of talking about him or doing him harm in some way. Although he liked his job and was successful in it, he sometimes found it very difficult to go to work. All his sexual contacts were with casual partners he met in cruising areas, since he was too anxious to show that he might like to meet someone and certainly too anxious to pick anyone up. He had had multiple casual partners with whom he mostly engaged in unprotected oral sex but also unprotected active and passive intercourse. He had been tested for HIV antibodies six times in the last two years. Because of his mood, he had gone out very little in recent weeks and reported only one incident of unprotected intercourse in the previous three months, although in more normal circumstances, he would be having up to six sexual contacts per month.

He described himself as having no confidence and said he had felt depressed for a long time. In fact, he had consulted a psychiatrist in Spain two years previously, who prescribed antidepressants, and again in London one year previously, who again prescribed antidepressants and referred him to the substance misuse service because of his polydrug use. He did not take the prescribed medication for long, because he found it increased his anxiety. He had managed to reduce his recreational drug use but still drank a good deal of alcohol, scoring above the cut-off for problem drinking on the CAGE. His score on the neuroticism dimension of the EPQ-R was more than twice the average for his age group and he also had a very high score on the GHQ-28, confirming a considerable degree of psychological distress. He had insight into his unsafe sexual behaviour saying that he was risky 'when I don't feel good about myself' and recognized that his self-imposed restriction to casual partners was motivated by a fear of rejection. Some of the remarks he made illustrate his beliefs about himself:

- I'm always in the wrong place at the wrong time.
- If people at home and my family knew [about his sexuality], they would reject me.
- Others are better than me.
- He is not the type of person who would want to talk to me.
- If someone gives me a compliment, I think, Why are they saying that?.
- I'll be alone all my life.
- Nobody can be trusted.

Gradually, he revealed some of the origins of his beliefs. His cultural and religious upbringing was one in which homosexuality was never discussed, and he grew up with the feeling that it was totally unacceptable. An incident in early childhood in which a teacher reprimanded him in a very public manner for playing with another boy left him feeling confused and humiliated. Later, as a young teenager, he had regular sexual contacts with a close friend for six years. The friend married at 20 and never spoke of their relationship again. When FD came to England, he fell in love and believed it was reciprocated, but later found out that his lover was married with two children. He felt betrayed by both these relationships and found it impossible to trust anyone as a consequence. Even so, he blamed himself for the break-up of the relationships and this gave a clue to his core beliefs about himself, expressed in the feeling that he was not as good as others.

Treatment

By using cognitive therapy approaches such as the downward arrow technique, in which the person is guided to discovering the thoughts underlying statements such as 'I don't deserve any better' by a series of questions, FD found that his core schema was 'The way I am is not acceptable'. This was helpful in explaining his automatic thoughts about people looking at him and criticizing him. It also helped to explain his anxiety in social situations and his unsafe sexual behaviour. The most salient automatic thoughts associated with unsafe sex identified by the SRCQ were 'I want to show him he is special' and 'I feel pressured not to use a condom'. FD also recognized that when he was drunk, he would think 'Who cares: life is a risk' and 'I can do what I like' – expressions of feeling in control at the time. The formulation in Figure 10.3 was agreed with FD and formed the basis for the intervention.

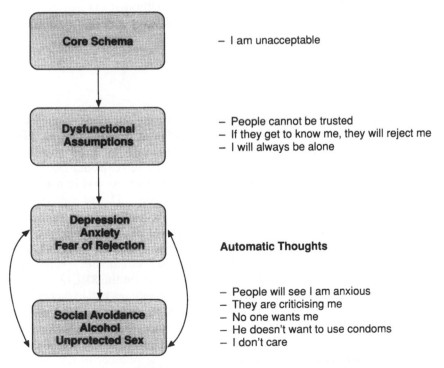

Figure 10.3 *Formulation for FD.*

Once the core belief was identified, various approaches, including continuum methods and self-questioning, were used to help FD reappraise his damaging belief. During seven treatment sessions over a period of five months, he learned to question his thoughts instead of perceiving them as facts, so he was able to say by the end of treatment, 'No-one is superior: we are all the same, some good parts and some not so good' and 'I deserve better: I am as good as anyone else'. He also successfully challenged the thoughts which made unsafe sex more likely, principally by developing positive statements about condom use, such as 'Condoms are cleaner', 'They don't stop me enjoying the sex', 'I prefer to use a condom, I am in control'. He also began routinely keeping condoms accessible.

Another aspect of treatment concerned his extreme social anxiety and panic attacks. Although he began to feel better about himself through practice in thought challenging, he needed to overcome his avoidance of crowded places and public transport. He particularly wanted to be able to go to clubs and other venues in which he might have the opportunity of meeting a partner and had set himself the goal of stopping casual sexual encounters in cruising areas. A graded exposure programme was agreed. He began by attending a party which was difficult for him. Although he was very anxious, he coped rather better than he had expected, and this greatly increased his confidence in being able to deal with other social situations. Soon he was able to go to a club alone and even to meet a sexual partner there. Although FD had difficulty in resisting coercion to have unprotected sex, he showed with the condom demonstrator that he was skilled in condom use.

Outcome

During the course of the intervention FD began going out more, something he had been avoiding, as well as having more frequent sexual contacts. He recorded 12 episodes of active and passive intercourse in three months, all protected, including one encounter in which he resisted considerable pressure from his partner to be unsafe. Only one of these contacts was in his habitual cruising location. Three months after intervention, FD was still reporting consistent condom use in every encounter and his confidence in maintaining safer sex had increased from a pretreatment level of 2 to 4, where 6 is the maximum. The most striking changes were in his scores on the CAGE and GHQ-28, both of which had dropped to zero from pretreatment levels of 3 and 19, respectively. He also markedly reduced his score on the SRCQ from 77 to 37, supporting the idea that his cognitions about unsafe sex had in fact changed.

This case is one in which risk reduction skills training would not have been effective, since FD's core belief about his unacceptability was the driving force for his unhappiness, anxiety, alcohol use and unsafe sex. It also illustrates the way in which frequency of sexual behaviour or number of partners does not always reflect positive changes, since FD had only one sexual encounter in the three months before intervention, whereas after intervention his sexual activity increased as his mood and attitudes changed.

One of the main difficulties in evaluating the effectiveness of the intervention is the fact that the important outcome measures of sexual behaviour and confidence in the ability to maintain safer sex are necessarily self-reported. These outcome measures are backed up by inspection of the HIV/GUM database for each person seen, but absence of evidence of new STDs or of HIV seroconversion is not conclusive: many individuals are not consistent attenders at a particular clinic and may present at clinics in other parts of London. This appears to be particularly the case among HIV-infected gay men. Even 'hard' evidence may not be as useful as it seems. Some of the clients are referred precisely because of their anxieties about recent risk behaviour, and some are still in the window period when an HIV test will not reliably detect infection. Even if their behaviour changes, they may subsequently test positive because of risk behaviour before intervention.

On average, self-reported frequency of unprotected intercourse is reduced from almost half of all occasions to less than one-quarter, and the proportion reporting unsafe sex on every occasion from 33 to 11 per cent following intervention. Confidence in the ability to maintain safer sex increases and the proportion endorsing the 'completely confident' pole of the self-efficacy scale rises from 6 per cent before treatment to 40 per cent afterwards. Several studies indicate that self-efficacy about the ability to be safe predicts low risk sexual behaviour (Aspinwall *et al.*, 1991; De Wit *et al.*, 1996) and perceived behavioural control is an independent predictor of condom use (Godin *et al.*, 1996). Data on frequency of clinic visits for acute STDs were available for 19 individuals who had pre- and post-treatment clinic visits recorded on the HIV/GUM database. The mean number of STD infections per year was significantly reduced from 0.90 before to 0.19 after intervention.

In so far as the evaluation measures are adequate to assess effectiveness, the clinical intervention appears to reduce self-reported risk behaviour, increase confidence in the ability to maintain safer sex and reduce the frequency of new STDs. Levels of psychological morbidity are also significantly reduced.

Cost-effectiveness

The difficulties encountered in achieving referrals and the relatively low numbers who complete intervention have led us to question the value and cost-effectiveness of the clinical service. A formal cost analysis has not been carried out, but a number of points can be made. A generous estimate of the time spent by the clinical psychologists on risk reduction activities amounts to five sessions per week, so the total costs are about £20,000 a year, including overheads and costs of publicity materials. A recent article reviewing economic evaluation of HIV prevention initiatives states:

> An HIV prevention program is cost saving if the cost per HIV infection averted is less than roughly \$485,000–\$515,000. . . . Clearly, other intangible factors (e.g. pain and suffering) would raise this monetary valuation if they could be quantified. Also, survey methods used to assess a person's willingness-to-pay to avoid certain health hazards have generally yielded much higher valuations of human life. (Holtgrave, Quails and Graham, 1996, pp. 471–72)

The monetary value alone translates to over £300,000. This estimate was made before the introduction of the newer triple antiretroviral combination therapies which cost between £15,000 and £20,000 per person per year, although there may be some savings in terms of productivity and benefits if the promise of the treatments is fulfilled. A recent study of the cost-effectiveness of an HIV prevention skills training intervention for gay men concluded that not only was the intervention effective in reducing risk behaviour, it was also cost saving (Pinkerton, Holtgrave and Valdisserri, 1997). If our intervention has been successful in preventing only one person from being infected in the whole five-year period that the service has been offered, costs will have been saved.

As well as the clients who complete intervention, there are many who only attend for one or two sessions but this could still have provided some impetus for change. Even if change to consistent condom use in every sexual encounter is not achieved, a decrease in the proportion of unprotected encounters is a legitimate treatment goal. Pinkerton and Abramson (1996) show that occasional condom use can significantly reduce the risk of HIV infection under most HIV prevalence and infectivity conditions. Because the prevalence of HIV infection in London is higher than in the rest of the United Kingdom, and particularly high among gay men, the likelihood that those attending the service are at high risk is increased and the cost-effectiveness of facilitating even small positive changes in risk behaviour is enhanced.

Group interventions have not proved appropriate for the population referred for risk reduction, partly because the numbers referred are low but also because of the nature of the presenting psychological and behavioural difficulties, among which the issue of safer sex is often one of many problems. The individuals who take up the service are clearly different from those who took part in the successful cognitive-behavioural interventions described by Kelly *et al.* (1989, 1990). The participants in the Kelly *et al.* studies were volunteers and the groups took place at an earlier stage of the epidemic, when there was a particularly strong movement among gay men faced with the possibility of AIDS to mobilize resources to meet the threat.

Extraordinary changes in sexual behaviour among gay men were documented at the time the Kelly *et al.* studies were carried out. One could speculate that many people with the personal and emotional resources to effect sexual behaviour change were able to do so when the information about transmission became widely known. Those experiencing difficulties now may represent a much more vulnerable and heterogeneous population, including young people who have matured in the post-AIDS era as well as older individuals who have been resistant to safer-sex messages. We would also argue that group interventions are not likely to be useful among some sectors of the population in which HIV infection has been well established for many years, such as among gay men in urban areas.

The individuals we see for risk reduction are in no way representative of gay men in general nor of gay men attending HIV/GUM clinics. Many people choose to have unprotected sex in some situations with some partners. We are only concerned with those who are troubled by their behaviour and who have found it difficult to be as safe as they would like to be.

Of course, wider community-level approaches are essential to achieve large-scale changes in attitudes and social norms about safer sex, but it is important to have multiple strategies and not to fail the perhaps minority subgroup who have many difficulties and who can be helped by an intensive individual approach.

Acknowledgement

We wish to thank the risk reduction service attenders.

References

ASPINWALL, L.G., KEMENY, M.E., TAYLOR, S.E., SCHNEIDER, S.G. and DUDLEY, J.P. (1991) 'Psychosocial predictors of gay men's AIDS risk reduction behaviour', *Health Psychology*, **10**, pp. 432–44.

BECK, A.T. (1976) *Cognitive Therapy for the Emotional Disorders*, New York: International Universities Press.

CAHILL, C., LLEWELLYN, S.P. and PEARSON, C. (1991) 'Long-term effects of sexual abuse which occurred in childhood: a review', *British Journal of Clinical Psychology*, **30**, pp. 117–30.

CATCHPOLE, M.A., MERCEY, D.E., NICOLL, A., ROGERS, P.A., SIMMS, I., NEWHAM, J., MAHONEY, A., PARRY, J.V., JOYCE, C. and GILL, O.N. (1996) 'Continuing transmission of sexually transmitted diseases among patients infected with HIV-1 attending genitourinary medicine clinics in England and Wales', *British Medical Journal*, **312**, pp. 539–42.

CHOI, K. and COATES, T.J. (1994) 'Prevention of HIV infection', *AIDS*, **8**, pp. 1371–89.

COATES, T.J., AGGLETON, P., GUTZWILLER, F., DES JARLAIS, D., KLHARA, M., KIPPAX, S., SCHECTER, M. and VAN DEN HOEK, J.A.R. (1996) 'HIV prevention in developed countries', *Lancet*, **348**, pp. 1143–48.

COMMUNICABLE DISEASE REPORT (1998) 'AIDS and HIV infection in the United Kingdom: monthly report', *CDR*, **8**, 4, pp. 37–40.

COSTA, P.T. and MCRAE, R.R. (1992) *Revised NEO Personality Inventory (NEO-PI-R) and NEO Five Factor Inventory (NEO-FFI) Professional Manual*, Odessa FL: Psychological Assessment Resources.

DE WIT, J., HOSPERS, H., JANSSEN, M., STROEBE, W. and KOK, G. (1996) 'Risk for HIV infection among young gay men: sexual relations, high risk behaviour and protection motivation', paper presented at the Eleventh International Conference on AIDS, Vancouver, Canada.

DICLEMENTE, R.J., PIES, C.A., STOLLER, E.J., STRAITS, C., OLIVIA, G.E. and RUTHERFORD, G.W. (1989) 'Evaluation of school-based AIDS education curricula in San Francisco', *Journal of Sex Research*, **26**, pp. 188–98.

DI FRANCEISCO, W., OSTROW, D.G. and CHMIEL, J.S. (1996) 'Sexual adventurism, high-risk behaviour and human immunodeficiency virus-1 seroconversion among the MACS-CCS cohort, 1984–1992', *Sexually Transmitted Diseases*, **23**, pp. 453–60.

EKSTRAND, M.L., STALL, R.D., MARLATT, G.A., POLLACK, L.M. and MCKUSICK, L. (1992) 'Will the real relapsers please stand up?', paper presented at the Eighth International Conference on AIDS, Amsterdam.

ELLIS, D., COLLIS, I. and KING, M. (1994) 'A controlled comparison of HIV and general medical referrals to a liaison psychiatry service', *AIDS Care*, **6**, pp. 69–76.

ELLIS, D., COLLIS, I. and KING, M. (1995) 'Personality disorder and risk taking among homosexually active and heterosexually active men attending a genitourinary medicine clinic', *Journal of Psychosomatic Research*, **39**, pp. 901–10.

EVANS, B.G., CATCHPOLE, M.A., HEPTONSTALL, J., MORTIMER, J.Y., MCCARRIGLE, C.A., NICOLL, A.G., WAIGHT, P., GILL, O.N. and SWAN, A.V. (1993) 'Sexually transmitted diseases and HIV-1 infection among homosexual men in England and Wales', *British Medical Journal*, **306**, pp. 426–28.

EYSENCK, H.J. and EYSENCK, S.B.G. (1991) *Manual of the Eysenck Personality Scales*, London: Hodder and Stoughton.

GODIN, G., SAVARD, J., KOK, G., FORTIN, C. and BOYER, R. (1996) 'HIV seropositive gay men: understanding adoption of safe sexual practices', *AIDS Education and Prevention*, **8**, pp. 529–45.

GOLD, R.S. and ROSENTHAL, D.A. (1995) 'Preventing unprotected anal intercourse in gay men: a comparison of two intervention techniques', *International Journal of STD and AIDS*, **6**, pp. 89–94.

GOLD, R.S. and SKINNER, M.J. (1992) 'Situational factors and thought processes associated with unprotected intercourse in young gay men', *AIDS*, **6**, pp. 1021–30.

GOLD, R.S., SKINNER, M.J. and ROSS, M.W. (1994) 'Unprotected anal intercourse in HIV-infected and non-HIV-infected gay men', *Journal of Sex Research*, **31**, pp. 59–77.

GOLD, R.S., SKINNER, M.J., GRANT, P.J. and PLUMMER, D.C. (1991) 'Situational factors and thought processes associated with unprotected intercourse in gay men', *Psychology and Health*, **5**, pp. 259–78.

GOLDBERG, D.P. and HILLIER, V.F. (1979) 'A scaled version of the General Health Questionnaire', *Psychological Medicine*, **9**, pp. 139–45.

GRAY, D., BUTTON, J., SHAH, D. and BARTON, S. (1997) 'Failure to prevent HIV infection among gay men previously tested HIV negative', paper presented at AIDS Impact, The Third International Conference on Biopsychosocial Aspects of HIV Infection, Melbourne.

HATHAWAY, S.R. and MCKINLEY, J.C. (1989) *The Minnesota Multiphasic Personality Inventory Manual*, Minneapolis MN: National Computer Systems.

HAYS, R.B., PAUL, J., EKSTRAND, M., KEGELES, S.M., STALL, R. and COATES, T.J. (1997) 'Actual versus perceived HIV status, sexual behaviors and predictors of unprotected sex among young gay and bisexual men who identify as HIV-negative, HIV-positive and untested', *AIDS*, **11**, pp. 1495–1502.

HELMES, E. and REDDON, J.R. (1993) 'A perspective on developments in assessing psychopathology: a critical review of the MMPI and MMPI-2', *Psychological Bulletin*, **113**, pp. 453–71.

HOLTGRAVE, D.R., QUAILS, N.L. and GRAHAM, J.D. (1996) 'Economic evaluation of HIV prevention programs', *Annual Review of Public Health*, **17**, pp. 467–88.

HURLEY, S.F., JOLLEY, D.J. and KALDOR, J.M. (1997) 'Effectiveness of needle exchange programmes for prevention of HIV infection', *Lancet*, **349**, pp. 1797–1800.

JEMMOTT, J.D., JEMMOTT, L.S. and FONG, G.T. (1992) 'Reductions in HIV risk-associated sexual behaviours among black male adolescents: effects of an AIDS prevention intervention', *American Journal of Public Health*, **82**, pp. 372–77.

JINICH, S., PAUL, J.P., STALL, R., ACREE, M., KEGELES, S., HOFF, C. and COATES, T.J. (1998) 'Childhood sexual abuse and HIV risk-taking sexual behaviour among gay and bisexual men', *AIDS and Behaviour*, **2**, pp. 41–52.

KALICHMAN, S.C., CAREY, M.P. and JOHNSON, B.T. (1997) 'Prevention of sexually transmitted HIV infection: a meta-analytic review of the behavioural outcome literature', *Annals of Behavioural Medicine*, **18**, pp. 6–15.

KALICHMAN, S.C., JOHNSON, J.R., ADAIR, V., ROMPA, D., MULTHAUF, K. and KELLY, J.A. (1994) 'Sexual sensation seeking: scale development and predicting AIDS-risk behaviour among homosexually active men', *Journal of Personality Assessment*, **62**, pp. 385–97.

KALICHMAN, S.C., KELLY, J.A., MORGAN, M. and ROMPA, D. (1997) 'Fatalism, current life satisfaction, and risk for HIV infection among gay and bisexual men', *Journal of Consulting and Clinical Psychology*, **65**, pp. 542–46.

KELLY, J.A. (1995) 'Advances in HIV/AIDS education and prevention', *Family Relations*, **44**, pp. 345–52.

KELLY, J.A., ST LAWRENCE, J.D., HOOD, H.V. and BRASFIELD, T.L. (1989) 'Behavioural intervention to reduce AIDS risk activities', *Journal of Consulting and Clinical Psychology*, **57**, pp. 60–67.

KELLY, J.A., ST LAWRENCE, J.D., BETTS, R., BRASFIELD, T.L. and HOOD, H.V. (1990) 'A skills-training group intervention model to assist persons in reducing risk behaviours for HIV infection', *AIDS Education and Prevention*, **2**, pp. 24–35.

KIPPAX, S., CRAWFORD, J., DAVIS, M., RODDEN, P. and DOWSETT, G. (1993) 'Sustaining safer sex: a longitudinal study of homosexual men', *AIDS*, **7**, pp. 257–63.

KIRBY, D., BARTH, R.P., LELAND, N. and FERRO, J.D. (1991) 'Reducing the risk: impact of a new curriculum on sexual risk-taking', *Family Planning Perspectives*, **23**, pp. 253–63.

KLINE, P. (1993) *The Handbook of Psychological Testing*, London: Routledge.

MCKIRNAN, D.J., OSTROW, D.G. and HOPE, B. (1996) 'Sex, drugs and escape: a psychological model of HIV-risk behaviours', *AIDS Care*, **6**, pp. 655–69.

MAYFIELD, D., MCLEOD, G. and HALL, P. (1974) 'The Cage questionnaire: validation of a new alcoholism screening instrument', *American Journal of Psychiatry*, **131**, pp. 1121–23.

MEYER, R.G. (1993) *The Clinician's Handbook: Integrated Diagnosis, Assessment and Intervention in Adult and Adolescent Psychopathology*, Needham Heights MA: Allyn & Bacon.

MILLER, E., WAIGHT, R.S., TEDDER, R.S., SUTHERLAND, S., MORTIMER, P.P. and SHAFI, M.S. (1995) 'Incidence of HIV infection in homosexual men in London, 1988–94', *British Medical Journal*, **311**, p. 545.

OAKLEY, A., FULLERTON, D. and HOLLAND, J. (1995) 'Behavioural interventions for HIV/AIDS prevention', *AIDS*, **9**, pp. 479–86.

OSMOND, D., PAGE, A., WILEY, J., GARRETT, K., SHEPPARD, H., MOSS, A., SCHRAGER, L. and WINKELSTEIN, W. (1994) 'Human immunodeficiency virus infection in homosexual and bisexual men, 18 to 29 years of age: the San Francisco young men's health study', *American Journal of Public Health*, **84**, pp. 1933–37.

OTTEN, M.W., ZAIDI, A.A., WROTEN, J., WITTE, K. and PETERMAN, T. (1993) 'Changes in sexually transmitted disease rates after HIV testing and post-test counselling, Miami, 1988–1989', *American Journal of Public Health*, **83**, pp. 529–33.

PADESKY, C.A. (1994) 'Schema change processes in cognitive therapy', *Clinical Psychology and Psychotherapy*, **1**, pp. 267–78.

PADESKY, C.A. (1995) 'Schema as self-prejudice', *International Cognitive Therapy Newsletter*, **5/6**, pp. 16–17. Available from K. Mooney (ed.), Centre for Cognitive Therapy, 1101 Dove Street, Suite 240, Newport Beach, CA 92660, USA.

PERKINS, D.O., DAVIDSON, E.J., LESERMAN, J., LIAO, D. and EVANS, D.L. (1994) 'Personality disorder in patients infected with HIV: a controlled study with implications for clinical care', *American Journal of Psychiatry*, **150**, pp. 309–15.

PINKERTON, S.D. and ABRAMSON, P.R. (1996) 'Occasional condom use and HIV risk reduction', *Journal of Acquired Immunodeficiency Syndromes and Human Retrovirology*, **13**, pp. 456–60.

PINKERTON, S.D., HOLTGRAVE, D.R. and VALDISSERRI, R.O. (1997) 'Cost-effectiveness of HIV-prevention skills training for men who have sex with men', *AIDS*, **11**, pp. 347–57.

RIDGE, D. (1996) 'Negotiated safety: not negotiable or safe?', *Venereology*, **9**, pp. 98–100.

ROSENBERG, P.S. (1994) 'Backcalculation models of age-specific HIV incidence rates', *Statistical Medicine*, **13**, pp. 1975–90.

ROTHERAM-BORUS, M.J., KOOPMAN, C., HAIGNERE, C. and DAVIES, M. (1991) 'Reducing HIV risk behavior among runaway adolescents', *Journal of the American Medical Association*, **266**, pp. 1237–41.

SCRAGG, P. (1995) *Psych D portfolio*, University of Surrey.

SCRAGG, P., SHAH, D. and THORNTON, S. (in press) 'Personality traits among individuals who have problems with safer sex'.

SHAH, D., THORNTON, S. and BURGESS, A. (1997) 'The sexual risk cognitions questionnaire: a reliability and validity study', *AIDS Care*, **9**, pp. 471–80.

SHARP, R., CROFTS, N., SATTLER, G., MARCUS, L. MAEDE, J., WALLACE, J. and WOOD, R. (1996) 'Negotiated safety? Sexual practices among young gay injecting drug users', *Venereology*, **9**, pp. 106–12.

STALL, R. and EKSTRAND, M. (1994) 'The quantitative/qualitative debate over 'relapse' behaviour: comment', *AIDS Care*, **6**, pp. 619–24.

STRATHDEE, S.A., HOGG, R.S., MARTINDALE, S.L., CORNELISSE, P.G.A., CRAIB, K.J.P., SCHILDER, A., MONTANER, J.S.G., O'SHAUGHNESSY, M.V. and SCHECTER, M.T. (1996) 'Sexual abuse is an independent predictor of sexual risk taking among young HIV-negative gay men: results from a prospective study', paper presented at the Eleventh International Conference on AIDS, Vancouver.

TALLIS, F. (1995) 'Cognitive behavioural strategies for HIV sexual risk reduction', *Clinical Psychology and Psychotherapy*, **1**, pp. 267–77.

THORNTON, S., TALLIS, F., FLYNN, R., CATALÁN, J. and ARONEY, R. (1994) 'Applying the cognitive behavioural model to interventions for HIV sexual risk reduction', paper presented at AIDS Impact, The Second International Conference on Biopsychosocial Aspects of HIV Infection, Brighton.

UNAIDS/WHO (1997) *Report of the Working Group on Global HIV/AIDS and STD Surveillance*.

WALTER, H.J. and VAUGHAN, R.D. (1993) 'Aids risk reduction among a multi-ethnic sample of Cuban high school students', *Journal of the American Medical Association*, **270**, pp. 725–30.

WELLINGS, K., WADSWORTH, J., JOHNSON, A.M., FIELD, J., WHITAKER, L. and FIELD, B. (1995) 'Provision of sex education and early sexual experience: the relation examined', *British Medical Journal*, **311**, pp. 417–20.

YOUNG, J. (1990) *Cognitive therapy for personality disorders: a schema-focused approach*, Sarasota FL: Professional Resource Exchange.

ZENILMAN, J., ERICKSON, B., FOX, R., REICHART, C. and HOOK, E. (1992) 'Effect of HIV post-test counselling on STD incidence', *Journal of the American Medical Association*, **267**, pp. 843–45.

Chapter 11

Psychoneuroimmunology and HIV Infection

Simon Dupont and Adrian Burgess

The study of the relationship between psychological factors and bodily health is a long-standing one, including a wide range of physical disorders and psychological variables. HIV disease is no exception, and there has been considerable interest in the relationship between mood, stress and other variables and their effect on disease progression and survival. In this chapter the general relationship between psychological factors and health is reviewed, with emphasis on empirical research and experiments that have focused on psychological and personality factors in HIV infection.

What is Psychoneuroimmunology?

Psychoneuroimmunology is the study of how the mind influences the development or progression of physical disease. At present, one of the main aims of psychoneuroimmunology is to establish whether there is an association between psychological factors and immunological function. For example, can depression, anxiety or psychological distress alter our ability to resist infection, autoimmune diseases, or cancer? If so, can we alter immunological function and hence susceptibility to disease through psychological interventions? Although it is impossible to answer these questions categorically at the present time, there is a growing body of research focusing on such issues.

Psychological Factors Influencing Health Status

Figure 11.1 presents a summary of how psychological factors might alter immunological functioning susceptibility to disease (Cohen and Herbert, 1996). Psychological factors may influence immunological function through direct innervation of the CNS (e.g. changing the rate of flow of cytokines across the blood–brain barrier). Alternatively, immunological function may be influenced via the endocrine system (e.g. hormone levels are known to be affected by psychological factors such as chronic stress). Finally, behaviour may have important influences on the development and progression of disease. This may include lifestyle (diet, exercise, substance use) as well as behavioural changes influenced by personality, affect or ways of coping with stressful events. Re-

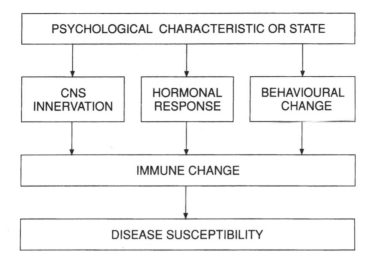

Figure 11.1 *How psychological factors might influence the onset and progression of diseases mediated by the immune system. Adapted from Cohen and Herbert (1996).*

search into the psychological factors that may be important influences on immunological function can be categorized into four main areas: affect, stress, interpersonal relationships and personality. Each will be discussed in turn before looking more closely at psychological factors and HIV infection.

Affect

A large number of studies have focused on clinical depression when investigating the role of affect in immune response. Depression is associated with an increased risk to physical morbidity and mortality, and changes in affect produce immune system responses (Ader, Felten and Cohen, 1991). A meta-analysis of over 40 studies shows that, compared to healthy controls, clinically depressed individuals have lowered numbers of NK, B, T, and helper T cells, and lowered lymphocyte activity (Herbert and Cohen, 1993). As will be discussed under methodology, the relationship between depression and immunological function might be mediated by behavioural factors. Depressed persons sleep less, exercise less, have poorer diets, smoke more and use alcohol and drugs more often than non-depressed persons (Gregory and Smeltzer, 1983). It is difficult, therefore, to establish whether depression per se causes changes in immunological function or whether it is moderating behavioural factors.

Stress

Probably the most well-known set of studies of stress and immunological function are by Kiecolt-Glaser *et al.* (1984, 1986), Glaser *et al.* (1985, 1987,

1991, 1993) with the impact of medical school examinations in medical students' cellular immunological function. Medical students showed a decrease in the function of a range of indicators of cellular immune response, including decreased NK activity, lymphocyte proliferation and production, as well as increase in production of antibody to herpes viruses.

The effects of chronic stress have also been investigated. Residents surrounding the Three Mile Island nuclear power plant showed lower cellular immune competence which was not due to radiation (total T lymphocyte, T4 and macrophage cell numbers) than in demographically matched controls almost ten years after the accident (McKinnon *et al.*, 1989).

Interpersonal Relationships

Substantial evidence implicates interpersonal relationships in the maintenance of health (Cohen, 1988; House, Landis and Umberson, 1988). Glaser *et al.* (1985) found that medical students reporting high levels of loneliness had lower NK activity and higher levels of herpes virus antibody than those who described themselves as less lonely. Poorer marital relations and marital disruption are associated with poorer health (Verbrugge, 1979) and perceived availability of social support has also been associated with immunological function.

Personality

Much has been written about personality and health, particularly in relation to heart disease. The general consensus seems to be that hostility is the critical factor in heart disease (Barefoot, 1992). However, relations between personality characteristics and immunological function have received little attention. Hislop *et al.* (1987) found greater survival from breast cancer among women high on extraversion and low in anger. Neuroticism was shown to be related to recurrent urinary tract infection (Hunt and Waller, 1992).

Psychoneuroimmunology and HIV Infection

The discussion so far has focused on the associations between psychological factors and immunological function among healthy individuals. Another burgeoning body of research looks at psychological factors among people who are suffering from a particular disease, such as cancer, arthritis or HIV. Within this area, studies can be divided into those investigating associations (including cross-sectional and longitudinal studies) and those investigating the effects of psychological interventions on disease course.

Methodological Considerations

Before discussing the HIV studies in detail, it is important to point out some of the formidable methodological difficulties that need to be overcome in order to establish a clear link between psychological factors and immunological functioning. For example, psychological factors may influence individual susceptibility to infection, yet identifying and studying individuals who are likely to be exposed to HIV infection presents considerable practical and ethical problems. Generally, therefore, participants are recruited into a study at the point they attend for HIV testing, by which time their psychological states may have changed substantially.

Another important methodological problem is the influence of social and behavioural factors on immunological function. Substance abuse (drugs, alcohol, caffeine and tobacco), nutrition, sexual activity, aerobic fitness, sleep patterns, medication, social class, occupation and age may all affect both the immune system and an individual's psychological state (Ader, 1988; Goodkin, Fletcher and Cohen, 1995). For example, someone who is depressed is likely to have altered sleep patterns, eat poorly, be less active and may use more drugs and alcohol. They might also be less inclined to adhere to prescribed HIV medication. Another potential confounding variable is sexual behaviour. Psychological factors are related to the initiation and nature of sexual behaviour (Bancroft, 1989). Among HIV positive individuals, reinfection or exposure to other STDs due to unsafe sex, perhaps prompted by feelings of hopelessness or fatalism, may accelerate the course of HIV (Detels, English and Visscher, 1989; Phair, Jacobson and Detels, 1991). Therefore, what may appear to be a direct relationship between psychological factors and immune parameters may in fact be mediated by changes in health-related behaviours.

On a more practical level, there are no definitive measures of immunological function in psychoneuroimmunological research. The exact nature of any given immune response varies with the invaded organism's history of exposure, the type of antigen, and the route of entry into the body. Researchers are limited to assessing a small number of crude markers of immunological function rather than anything that resembles a true estimate of the body's ability to resist disease. The difficult question is determining the most appropriate measures of immunological function. The CD4 count has been used routinely in many studies of HIV infection because it is regularly taken and easily available. However, CD4 count might not be the most appropriate measure for psychoneuroimmunological research as it is relatively unreactive over the short term (Stein, Miller and Trestman, 1991) but may be more informative over longer periods.

Viral load testing measures the levels of HIV in the blood and therefore may give a more accurate indicator of HIV progression, yet only 2 per cent of HIV is in circulating blood, with the majority being in the lymph system and other body tissue. Another alternative involves measuring the response of different lymphocyte subsets such as lymphocyte proliferation to mitogen and natural killer cytotoxicity (NKCC). These measures may be more sensitive to psychological influences but are also more difficult, expensive and time-consuming to measure. An added complication is the natural diurnal variation in the CD4 cell count and NKCC. It is important that blood is taken from participants at the same time of day to limit this confounding variable.

The choice of psychological measures is also a difficult issue. By definition, state measures such as anxiety and depression are likely to change over time, so in general they do not have good predictive value longitudinally. More stable psychological characteristics such as personality, coping style and social support might need to be assessed in addition to measures of mood.

Cross-sectional studies enable associations to be identified; but in order to make predictions, longitudinal designs are needed. The length of the follow-up period for longitudinal studies is important in order to demonstrate meaningful changes in the dependent variable. Within HIV studies this time lag is critical, particularly as the majority of individuals with HIV may take three years before they show a significant reduction in CD4 levels (Detels *et al.*, 1988).

There are a variety of groups of individuals with HIV, including gay and bisexual men, children, intravenous drug users, heterosexuals, and men with haemophilia. Within each group, there are differences in ethnic background, gender and age. Risk group, age and ethnicity appear to be predictors of HIV progression rate (Gardner *et al.*, 1992; Rothenberg *et al.*, 1987; Munoz *et al.*, 1988). Consequently, these potential confounding variables need to be taken into account when analyzing results.

Research evidence in psychoneuroimmunology of HIV infection can be classified in three ways: the first involves cross-sectional design studies, the second involves longitudinal studies and the third examines the effect of specific interventions. Published studies from each of these three categories will be discussed.

Cross-sectional Studies

In order to study the relationship between mood state and immunological function, Sahs *et al.* (1994) looked at the psychological distress in 74 HIV positive and 46 HIV negative gay men. Comparisons were made between HIV negative, HIV positive asymptomatic and HIV positive symptomatic men by using a variety of clinician-rated and self-reported measures of psychological function and absolute natural killer (NK) cell number. Psychological measures included anxiety and depression, hopelessness, social support, symptom inventory and global functioning. They found that in the cohort of 120 gay men, NK cell counts were largely unrelated to psychological variables. Moreover, specific factors previously reported to predict decreased NK cells, such as depression, were not predictive for this group of men. Also, while HIV infection was associated with a significant decrease in NK cell number, HIV positive men were no more susceptible than HIV negative men to the deleterious effects of psychosocial distress on NK cells. In conclusion the authors state that 'No connection between psychology and immunological function was detected' (*ibid.*, p. 1482).

A cross-sectional study that did find a relationship between psychological factors and immunological function was conducted by Evans *et al.* (1995). Information about stressful life events and depression was obtained from 99 HIV positive and 65 HIV negative gay men using a semistructured interview. Immunological measures included numbers of NK cells, CD4 T cells and CD8 T cells. Results showed a clear relation between severe stress and reductions in killer lymphocytes (NK and CD8 cells) among the HIV sample. The relationship was not explained by confounding variables such as greater depression in participants with more stress, or by more advanced disease. In the HIV negative men no clear and consistent relation between stress and immunological functioning was found. Both studies were part of a much larger longitudinal investigation which will be discussed below.

The Evans *et al.* paper notes a clear association between stress and immunological function. Two of the known mediators of life stressors are social support and coping style. It is possible that the association between stress and immunological function is influenced by the support a person has and the coping strategies he uses. Social support is viewed as a protection, buffering the individual from the psychological consequences of the stressor (Cobb, 1976; Cassel, 1976). Different coping styles are viewed as adaptive or maladaptive to the stressful situation (Folkman and Lazarus, 1980) and many researchers are currently examining which strategies are most useful for dealing with particular stressors. As a follow-on from the Evans *et al.* study, Goodkin *et al.* (1992) investigated the association between coping style, social support and life stressors on the immunology of 62 HIV positive gay men. Control measures for alcohol/substance use and nutritional status were also included. They found a direct and positive association between an active coping style and natural killer cell cytotoxicity (NKCC), so that individuals using active coping as a strategy also had high NKCC. Decrements in NKCC are viewed as indicating a compromised immune system. Having active coping associated with higher NKCC levels may demonstrate the impact of psychological factors on the immune system. But as the study was cross-sectional, it holds no predictive power and conclusions concerning causality are therefore unsound. Other weaker and negative associations were found between both a passive coping style, life stresses and NKCC, which fits the psychoneuro-immunology model. A weak positive link was apparent between social support and NKCC, indicating the buffering effect of social support on life stressors.

In summary the evidence from cross-sectional studies is interesting but lacking in consistency (Table 11.1). There is a suggestion from some studies that psychosocial factors and immunological function are linked but more rigorous research is needed. We will now examine longitudinal studies involving HIV and the immune system.

Table 11.1 *Summary of cross-sectional research into the psychoneuroimmunology of HIV infection*

Authors/group	Design	Psychological measures	Immunological measures	Authors' conclusions
Evans *et al.* (1995) University of Florida	99 HIV positive (asymptomatic) and 65 HIV negative gay men Assessed cross-sectionally using a semistructured interview	Stressful life events (PERI) Hamilton depression rating scale Structured clinical interview (SCID-RDC) Cigarette smoking (0–6 scale)	Lymphocyte subtest counts Lymphocyte responsivity	Severe stress was significantly associated with reduction in natural killer cell population among HIV positive groups; this relationship was not explained by changes in depression or ill health No significant relationship was found among HIV negative groups between stress and immunity
Goodkin *et al.* (1992) University of Miami	62 HIV positive (asymptomatic) gay/bisexual men were assessed cross-sectionally	Life events (LES) Social support (SPS) Coping style (COPE) Mood states (POMS)	Natural killer cell responsivity	Active coping was positively associated with natural killer cell activity
Sahs *et al.* (1994) University of Columbia, New York	74 HIV positive and 46 HIV negative gay men	Brief symptoms inventory Structured clinical interview (SCID-RDC) Global assessment of functioning scale Hamilton anxiety and depression rating scales Beck hopelessness inventory Social support scale	Natural killer cell counts	Natural killer cell counts were unrelated to psychological variables, regardless of status of individual

Longitudinal Studies

Burack *et al.* (1993) examined depression and CD4 counts in 330 HIV seropositive gay men over a four-year period. They reported that individuals who were identified as clinically depressed at baseline had a 40 per cent greater decline in CD4+ cells over a four-year period than their non-depressed counterparts. This data indicates that clinical depression may accelerate HIV disease progression.

Broadening the study beyond depression, Vedhara *et al.* (1997) looked at anxiety, depression as well as the functional and emotional impact of stress on disease progression in 125 HIV seropositive gay men over 12 months. Their resulting 'emotional distress' score, along with CD4+ cell count at diagnosis, were significant independent predictors of CD4+ cell count 12 months later. The authors conclude that the study offers further support for the idea of a significant relationship between emotional distress and HIV progression.

Looking at one of the most stressful of life experiences, Kemeny *et al.* (1995) examined immune system changes after the death of an intimate partner in both HIV seropositive and HIV seronegative gay men and explored the relationship between depressed mood and immune changes. The bereaved group consisted of 39 gay men whose intimate partners had died of AIDS over the past year; the control group consisted of 39 non-bereaved men matched by age and HIV serostatus. The results showed that among the HIV seropositive men, immune change consistent with HIV progression occurred after bereavement, whereas the non-bereaved HIV seropositive comparison group exhibited no such change. The authors had hypothesized that changes in immune parameters after bereavement would be particularly evident in individuals with high levels of depressed mood. However, depressed mood was uncorrelated with immune parameters in the bereaved group. Among the non-bereaved group, higher levels of depressed mood were significantly correlated with immune processes relevant to HIV progression. The authors conclude that bereavement is associated with the progression of HIV but not through the most obvious mediator of depression, and they discuss the difference between grief and depression. For the non-bereaved, depression does appear to be associated with the progression of HIV.

These three studies all conclude in favour of psychological factors, particularly depression, influencing immunological function. Yet in contrast to what might appear to be a seemingly robust association between affect and HIV progression, Mayne *et al.* (1996) followed up a group of 402 HIV seropositive gay men over a maximum of eight years. They reported that the more frequently a participant had elevated depressive affect, the greater his risk of mortality. Yet, importantly, this association was independent of physiological and clinical measures of HIV disease progression, i.e. clinical depression had no influence on the progression of HIV.

Again, but in a much larger study, Lyketsos *et al.* (1993) reported that they failed to find a significant association between baseline depression scores and CD4+ decline, which was assessed over an 8-year period. The study consisted of 1,809 HIV seropositive gay/bisexual men who were assessed semi-annually using the CES-D depression scale. The disparity of results from this well-designed, large-scale study compared to the other studies cited above indicates the enormous difficulties in reaching any overall conclusion with regards to psychoneuroimmunology.

Other investigators have examined a wider range of psychological measures (including depression) and their impact on the immune system of HIV seropositive individuals. Perry *et al.* (1992) studied 221 HIV seropositive individuals of both sexes and mixed risk factors over a one-year period. Patients were assessed on 22 psychosocial variables, including degree of depression, anxiety, intrusive and avoidant thoughts about HIV, stressful life events, hardiness, social support, hopelessness, personality disorder, psychiatric symptoms, bereavement and clinical ratings of psychopathology and global functioning. The major finding from the study was the lack of relationship between the psychosocial variables and immunological measures (CD4 and CD8 counts).

A similar conclusion was reached by Rabkin *et al.* (1991), who assessed 124 HIV seropositive gay/bisexual men at baseline and 6-month follow-up. Psychological measures included depression, anxiety, demoralization, hopelessness, social conflict, grief and life events. Again, immunological measures were CD4 and CD8 cell counts, and no significant associations with the psychosocial measures were found. In a critique of the two studies, Stein, Miller and Trestman (1991) stated, 'Both of these reports . . . suggest that psychosocial factors . . . do not have a measurable or substantial effect on the immune system in relation to physical disorders, such as AIDS' (p. 171).

In an enterprising study design, Ironson *et al.* (1990) assessed changes in psychological and immunological functioning during five-week periods preceding and following notification of serostatus among 46 gay males taking the HIV antibody test. Their premise was that both the anticipation and notification of HIV test results, particularly if the result was positive, would have a detrimental effect on the immune system during this period. They cited the Three Mile Island study (McKinnon *et al.*, 1989) discussed above as evidence for the effect of stressful situations on immunological function.

Psychological measures included anxiety, intrusive thoughts and avoidant behaviours. Most individuals who tested positive to HIV displayed clinical levels of anxiety, intrusive thoughts and avoidant responses during the week of notification, but returned to their initial baseline levels within five weeks. Interestingly, these same individuals did not show any change in immunological function even though psychological functioning deteriorated. The authors suggest this dissociation may indicate the inability of HIV seropositive individuals to mount an immune response to potent psychosocial stressors (i.e. serostatus notification), because the viral contribution to immunological functioning overrides any influence of environmental stimuli.

A more fruitful area has been the differences in coping style on immunological function. The Goodkin *et al.* (1992) active coping study has been discussed above. In a similar but prospective study, Mulder *et al.* (1995) looked at coping style, stressful life events, social support, psychiatric symptoms and HIV disease progression in 51 HIV seropositive gay men over 12 months. After adjustment for baseline biomedical parameters and behavioural variables, results showed that active confrontation with HIV infection as a coping strategy was predictive of decreased clinical progression of HIV infection at one year follow-up. Active confrontation consisted of seeking support, actively trying to solve problems and not denying the infection. No associations between the psychosocial parameters and CD4 counts were found.

Ironson *et al.* (1994), in a follow-on from the 1990 serostatus notification study, looked at coping style at the time of HIV testing. They found that the use of denial and behavioural disengagement to cope with receiving news of an HIV positive diagnosis was predictive of lower CD4 counts at one-year follow-up (controlling for CD4 counts at entry to the study), and greater likelihood of progression to HIV-related symptoms and AIDS at two-year follow-up. Similar results were found by Antoni *et al.* (1995) among 48 newly tested gay/ bisexual men; denial and disengagement as ways of coping with a positive diagnosis were predictive of greater immunological impairment at one-year follow-up. Interestingly, the opposite was found among the HIV negative group; greater disengagement coping predicted less immune impairment at one-year follow-up. The authors conclude that 'coping strategies relate to immunologic status differentially for infected and non-infected risk group members' (p. 234).

One investigation that found both positive and negative effects of coping on immunological functioning was by Solano *et al.* (1993). In their study, 100 HIV seropositive participants of both sexes and mixed risk factors were assessed at baseline, at 6 months and at 12 months. The use of a coping strategy characterized as 'fighting spirit' – an optimistic attitude accompanied by a search for greater information about HIV – appeared to be associated with less development of HIV-related symptoms during one year, whereas an attitude of denial or repression was associated with more HIV-related symptoms.

The literature on coping style cited above all appears to indicate that denial and disengagement leads to a poor immunological outcome, whereas actively coping with the disease has a positive effect. However, one investigation goes against this general theme. Reed *et al.* (1994) found that 'realistic acceptance' as a coping strategy was a significant predictor of decreased, rather than the expected increased, survival time in 74 gay men diagnosed with AIDS. This effect was not accounted for by demographic, immune or behavioural factors. In trying to reconcile this anomalous finding, Ironson *et al.* (1994) postulated that 'realistic acceptance' could be viewed as either a coping style or a predominantly negative cognitive orientation (fatalism) about the future, and it would make sense that being fatalistic about the future might lead to decreased survival time.

This postulation was borne out in a recent study by Thornton *et al.* (submitted), who investigated the contribution of psychological factors to disease progression in HIV infection among a group of long-term infected individuals. In their study, 147 gay men who had been infected for an average of 8.6 years completed self-report measures of a range of psychological variables and were followed up clinically for up to 32 months. Results demonstrated no effects of personality, psychological morbidity, social support, life events, handedness or socio-economic status, but acceptance coping was a significant predictor of longer ARC-free or AIDS-free survival (ARC is AIDS-related complex). Biomedical variables (e.g. viral load) were predominant in predicting survival time. The authors cite the Reed *et al.* study and discuss the contrasting findings. According to Thornton *et al.*, their wording of the acceptance factor 'does not have the elements of resignation and fatalism apparent in the description of stoic acceptance' from the Reed *et al.* study (p. 14).

The disparity of results highlights the difficulties of definition with respect to coping. There is no standard way of assessing coping, and it is unclear whether coping is situation-specific or dispositional. Nonetheless, the general trend from these studies appears to be that active coping is beneficial and denial or disengagement is detrimental to immunological functioning.

The last study in this section examines causal attribution as a predictor of immune decline. Segerstrom *et al.* (1996) hypothesized that attributions (perceived causes of events) would affect CD4 decline and onset of AIDS, either directly or through associations with psychological states such as depression. They interviewed 86 HIV seropositive gay men about their experiences with HIV and took blood samples over an 18-month period. The more attributions for negative events were rated as being internal-characterological (i.e. something about oneself), the faster CD4 cell number declined following the interview. Examples included 'I lost a couple of friends because I am HIV positive' and ' I won't be able to have a relationship because I am HIV positive'. The implication is that perceiving negative events as being due to some internal self-characteristic rather than an external cause has a significant detrimental effect on immunological functioning in the long term. The authors, however, did not find a significant association between negative self-beliefs and psychological constructs such as depression, indicating that depression was not the mediator between negative internal attributions and immune changes.

In summary the advantages of longitudinally designed studies in psychoneuroimmunology research appear to be somewhat outweighed by the conflicting results obtained (Table 11.2). One might have hoped the uncertainty and tenuous results from cross-sectional studies could be dismissed by the more robust, predictive nature of longitudinal research. This hope has yet to be borne out. Interpreting the results conservatively, it would appear that psychosocial factors have minimal influence over immunological function. Of all the areas investigated, coping style exhibits greatest potential for linking

Table 11.2 *Summary of longitudinal studies into the psychoneuroimmunology of HIV infection*

Authors/groups	Design	Psychological measures	Immunological measures	Authors' conclusions
Antoni *et al.* (1995) University of Miami	48 gay/bisexual men were assessed 5 weeks prior to, and 5 weeks after serostatus notification and at 1-year follow-up	Coping style (COPE)	Lymphocyte subset counts Natural killer cell cytotoxicity	Among HIV positive subjects, disengagement coping strategies were associated with lower CD4 and CD8 cell counts and predicted the same at 1 year follow-up; HIV negative men showed the opposite pattern
Burack *et al.* (1993) University of California, San Francisco	330 HIV positive (non-AIDS) gay/bisexual men were assessed and followed up with semi-annual assessments up to 66 months	Depression (CES-D)	Rate of decline of CD4 count	Depression is associated with a more rapid decline in CD4 count
Ironson *et al.* (1990) University of Miami	46 well, gay/bisexual men were assessed at intervals in the 5 weeks prior to HIV-1 serostatus notification and the 5 weeks afterwards	Anxiety (STAI) Intrusive thoughts (IES)	Lymphocyte subset counts Lymphocyte responsivity Natural killer responsivity	There was a dissociation between psychological and immunological responses in the HIV positive but not the HIV negative groups
Ironson *et al.* (1994) University of Miami	81 well, gay/bisexual men were assessed at 5 weeks prior to, 5 weeks post and up to 2 years after HIV-1 serostatus notification	Anxiety (STAI) Impact of events (IES) Mood (POMS) Denial coping (COPE) Treatment adherence	Lymphocyte responsivity CD4 cell count	Among the HIV positive group, the use of denial to deal with diagnosis was the strongest and most consistent predictor for deterioration of immune status and disease progression

Table 11.2 *Continued*

Authors/groups	Design	Psychological measures	Immunological measures	Authors' conclusions
				The second and third variables related to disease progression were respectively distress at diagnosis and treatment adherence
Kemeny *et al.* (1995) MACS study, Los Angeles	39 (both HIV positive and negative) gay/bisexual men who had suffered a bereavement over the previous year were compared with 39 matched non-bereaved controls	Mood states (POMS)	Lymphocyte subset counts Lymphocyte responsivity Neopterin	Among the HIV positive men, immune change consistent with HIV progression occurred after bereavement; this did not occur in the non-bereaved HIV positive comparison group In the non-bereaved group, those reporting depressed mood showed lower CD4 counts and lower proliferation response to phytohemaglutinin (PHA)
Lyketsos *et al.* (1993) MACS study, all sites combined	1,809 HIV positive (non-AIDS) gay/bisexual men were assessed semi-annually for up to 8 years	Depression (CES-D)	Rates of decline of CD4	Depression was not significantly associated with a more rapid decline in CD4 count
Mayne *et al.* (1996) University of California, San Francisco	402 HIV positive gay/bisexual men were assessed semi-annually for up to 8 years or until death, whichever the sooner	Depression (CES-D)	CD4 lymphocyte counts Rates of decline of CD4	Depressive affect was associated with mortality risk, but no association with depression and immunological measures

Study	Sample	Measures	Immunological measure	Findings
Mulder *et al.* (1995) Rotterdam, Netherlands	51 HIV positive (non-AIDS) gay men were assessed twice in a 1-year period	Psychiatric symptoms (GHQ-30) HIV life events list HIV coping list Social support questionnaire	CD4 lymphocyte counts	'Active confrontation' coping with HIV infection predicted less clinical progression of HIV infection
Perry *et al.* (1992) Cornell University Medical College, New York	221 HIV positive (non-AIDS) patients of both sexes and mixed risk factors were assessed at baseline, at 6 months and at 1 year	Depression (BDI) Brief symptom inventory anxiety (STAI) Intrusive thoughts (IES) Social support (ISEL) Hardiness (HQ) Life events Personality disorder questionnaire + clinical ratings	CD4 and CD8 count	There were no significant associations between the psychological and immunological measures
Rabkin *et al.* (1991) University of Columbia, New York	124 HIV positive (non-AIDS) gay/bisexual men were assessed at baseline, and at 6-month follow-up	Hamilton anxiety and depression rating scales Demoralization Hopelessness Social conflict Grief Life events	CD4 and CD8 count	There were no significant associations between the psychological and immunological measures
Reed *et al.* (1994) MACS study, Los Angeles	74 gay/bisexual men with AIDS were assessed every 6 months for up to 2 years	Affects balance scale Index of well-being Rosenberg self-esteem scale Kaplessmen scale Ways-of-coping scale (Lazarus)	CD4 cell count	Realistic acceptance as a way of coping was a significant predictor of decreased survival time

Table 11.2 *Continued*

Authors/groups	Design	Psychological measures	Immunological measures	Authors' conclusions
Solano et al. (1993) Instituto Italiano di Medicina Sociale, Rome	100 HIV positive (asymptomatic) subjects of both sexes and mixed risk factors were assessed at baseline and at 6 and 12 month follow-ups.	Social support scale Hardiness scale UCLA loneliness scale Family attitudes questionnaire Coping strategies[a]	CD4 count	Denial and repression were negatively associated with CD4 count and fighting spirit positively Hardiness and social support, in interaction with baseline CD4, were also associated with CD4
Thornton et al. (in press) Chelsea and Westminster Hospital, London	147 long-term HIV-infected men were assessed and were followed up clinically for up to 32 months.	General health questionnaire COPE Life experiences survey Interpersonal social support evaluation list EPQ Handedness	CD4 cell count Viral load	Acceptance coping was a significant predictor of longer ARC-free or AIDS-free survival
Vedhara et al. (1997) University of Bristol, UK	125 HIV positive gay men were assessed at baseline and at 6 and 12 month follow-ups.	Anxiety/depression (Savage personality screening scale) Global measure of perceived stress Stressful life events questionnaire Health status questionnaire	CD4 cell count	Emotional distress was a significant predictor for rate of CD4 cell loss

[a] Coping strategies: fighting spirit, helplessness, hopelessness, denial, repression.

psychology and immunology, with active strategies being seen as 'healthier' than passive strategies for the HIV seropositive individual.

Intervention Studies

One stage on from the 'look and see' approach of both cross-sectional and longitudinal designs is to manipulate one variable and measure its effect on another variable. Intervention studies, if properly conducted, may resolve many of the methodological problems associated with the other designs described above. Yet, to date, only a small number of intervention studies in this area have been published, with mixed but promising results.

One study that found positive results is by LaPerriere *et al.* (1990, 1991). Fifty HIV seropositive and HIV seronegative gay men were randomly assigned to either aerobic training or to a no-intervention control group. Participants were assessed following the five-week training period and 72 hours before notification of serostatus, with one further assessment a week after notification. HIV seropositive controls showed an increase in anxiety and depression and a reduction in natural killer cells following serostatus notification. HIV seropositive exercisers showed no change and did not differ from the HIV seronegative group.

In a parallel study from this group, 47 HIV seropositive asymptomatic gay men were randomly assigned to either a cognitive-behavioural stress management condition or an assessment-only control group, using the same five-week period before notification of HIV status as the exercise study (Antoni *et al.*, 1991). The HIV seropositive participants who underwent the stress management showed significant increases in CD4 and natural killer cell counts, with no significant increases in depression after notification. In contrast, HIV seronegative participants showed increased depression and no change in CD4 and natural killer cell counts. These studies support the notion that stress management and relaxation interventions can modulate mood and some measures of immunological functioning in early HIV infection. But as always, it is important to keep an open mind as other studies are less conclusive.

One such study looked at a more severely ill group to see whether stress management again had beneficial effects (Lutgendorf *et al.*, 1997). Participants were 33 HIV seropositive symptomatic gay men assigned to either a ten-week cognitive-behavioural stress management group or a waiting list control. Results show that the intervention significantly reduced depression and anxiety in HIV seropositive symptomatic gay men compared with controls, but neither group displayed changes in CD4 or CD8 cell numbers. The authors speculate that the lack of change in CD4 or CD8 cell counts may be due to the more severely ill patient group.

Coates *et al.* (1989) also found no immunological or affective changes between intervention and control group. Their study involved a stress-reduction intervention package (including relaxation, stress management skills and health behaviours) over eight weeks with 64 HIV seropositive men and waiting list controls. Auerbach, Oleson and Solomon, (1992) found similar results from a study of 26 HIV seropositive gay men assigned to either eight weeks of training to increase active coping skills and reduce stress (via thermal biofeedback, guided imagery and hypnosis) or a waiting list control group. There were no differences in CD4 count between the treatment group and controls, but there were also no differences between the groups on the psychological measures.

In summary the evidence here is at best mixed in its support for a role of psychosocial interventions in the progression of HIV infection (Table 11.3). Although many of the methodological difficulties obscuring longitudinal research are not so apparent, even quite promising areas such as coping style do not appear to be facilitated by intervention studies.

Discussion

The main focus of this chapter has been the relationship between psychological factors and immunological function. There is a wealth of evidence demonstrating the influence of psychological factors on a healthy immune system. The more difficult task is to demonstrate the part psychosocial factors play in altering immunological function in immune-system-mediated diseases such as HIV. The main obstacles for successful psychoneuroimmunology research are methodological. So many confounding variables, systematic errors, and factors such as choice of immunological or psychological measures have to be taken into account in order to make the results generalizable. It is not surprising, therefore, that only a relatively small number of high quality studies have been published. Unfortunately, no consistent theme emerges from these studies regardless of their design (cross-sectional, longitudinal or intervention).

One cannot categorically assert, for instance, that being clinically depressed will lead to faster HIV progression, or that coping with HIV by taking direct action to get round a problem will slow the course of the disease. If there is an impact of psychosocial factors on an HIV seropositive individual's immune system, it is marginal and can be obscured by a variety of methodological or design characteristics. Perhaps the major problem in this area is the lack of a coherent theoretical model that can be used as a basis for generating hypotheses. Figure 11.1 gives a broad outline of the factors involved but does not provide a theory as such. Research, then, is not theory-driven, making it difficult to generalize from study to study.

Even if it were possible to be certain that psychological factors played a significant role in the progression of HIV disease, this conclusion would not be without its dangers. Attributing an individual's health and survival to their own mental state can, at worst, be simply a way of 'blaming the victim'. Telling those who live with HIV infection that they can keep healthy by maintaining a positive outlook implies the corollary that if they get ill, it is their own fault.

Table 11.3 *Group summary of intervention studies into the psychoneuroimmunology of HIV infection*

Authors/groups	Design	Psychological measures	Immunological measures	Author conclusions
Antoni *et al.* (1991) University of Miami	47 well, gay/bisexual men were randomly assigned to a cognitive behavioural stress management programme or a waiting list control, 5 weeks prior to notification of HIV serostatus and 5 weeks afterwards	Coping style (COPE) Anxiety (STAI) Mood states (POMS) Intrusive thoughts (IES)	Lymphocyte subset counts Lymphocyte subset responsivity Cortisol β-endorphin	HIV positive subjects who underwent a stress management course showed no significant increase in depression, but did show increases in CD4 and natural killer cell counts. Controls showed increased depression and no change in CD4 or natural killer cell counts
Auerbach, Oleson and Solomon (1992) Health Establishment, Institute of California	26 HIV positive asymptomatic gay/bisexual men were randomly allocated to 8-week behavioural intervention or to a waiting list control	Mood states (POMS) Depression (BDI) Personal views survey HIV distress inventory	CD4 count	There were no differences in CD4 count between the treatment group and control, but there were also no differences between the groups on psychological measures
Coates *et al.* (1989) University of California, San Francisco	64 HIV positive gay/bisexual men (excluding those on medication and those with specific opportunistic infections) were randomly	None reported	Lymphocyte subset count Natural killer cell responsivity	There were no differences between treatment group and control group in lymphocyte number or function

Table 11.3 *Group summary of intervention studies into the psychoneuroimmunology of HIV infection*

Authors/groups	Design	Psychological measures	Immunological measures	Author conclusions
	allocated to eight 2-hour sessions of stress management or to a waiting list control		Lymphocyte responsivity	
LaPerriere *et al.* (1990, 1991) University of Miami	50 HIV positive asymptomatic gay/bisexual men were randomly assigned to 5 weeks of aerobic training or to a waiting list control prior to serostatus notification	Anxiety (COPE) Mood state (POMS)	Lymphocyte subset counts	HIV positive controls showed increase in anxiety and depression, and a reduction in natural killer cells following serostatus notification HIV positive exercisers showed no changes and did not differ from the HIV negative group
Lutgendorf *et al.* (1997) University of Miami	33 HIV positive symptomatic gay men were randomly allocated to 10-week cognitive behavioural stress management (CBSM) intervention of a modified waiting list control group	Depression (BDI) Mood states (POMS)	Lymphocyte subset counts Herpes simplex virus (HSV) types 1 and 2	Neither group displayed changes in CD4 or CD8 cell number or HSV-type 1 antibody titres. Individuals in CBSM had significantly decreased self-reported dysphoria, anxiety and total distress. The intervention also decreased HSV type 2 antibody titres

This 'tyranny of positive thinking' places an unreasonable burden on those with HIV infection and quite simply is not supported by the evidence. A positive outlook on life and an active coping style may be desirable in their own rights, but they probably have little, if any, effect on long-term survival in HIV disease.

Yet one must not lose sight of the original aims, namely to discover new ways of dealing with the virus and improving the patient's quality of life. Even though there might not be a link between affect and immunological function, treating someone's depression will undoubtedly increase their quality of life. Increasing a person's ability to cope with problems by teaching them new strategies might have major ramifications on their esteem, value and worth, even in the face of increasing HIV progression.

References

ADER, R. (1988) *Psychoneuroimmunology*, 2nd edn, San Diego CA: Academic Press.

ADER, R., FELTEN, D.L. and COHEN, N. (eds) (1991) *Psychoneuroimmunology*, New York: Academic Press.

ANTONI, M.H., BAGGETT, L., IRONSON, G., LaPERRIERE, A., AUGUST, S., KLIMAS, N., SCHNEIDERMAN, N. and FLETCHER, M. (1991) 'Cognitive-behavioural stress management intervention buffers distress responses and immunologic changes following notification of HIV-1 seropositivity', *Journal of Consulting and Clinical Psychology*, **59**, pp. 906–15.

ANTONI, M.H., GOLDSTEIN, D., IRONSON, G., LaPERRIERE, A., FLETCHER, M.A. and SCHNEIDERMAN, N. (1995) 'Coping responses to HIV-1 serostatus notification predict concurrent and prospective immunologic status', *Clinical Psychology and Psychotherapy*, **2**, pp. 234–48.

AUERBACH, J., OLESON, T. and SOLOMON, G. (1992) 'A behavioural medicine intervention as an adjuvant treatment for HIV-related illness', *Psychology and Health*, **6**, pp. 325–34.

BANCROFT, J. (1989) *Human Sexuality and its Problems*, 2nd edn, Edinburgh: Churchill Livingstone.

BAREFOOT, J.C. (1992) 'Developments in the measurement of hostility', in Friedman, H.S. (ed.) *Hostility, Coping and Health*, Washington DC: American Psychological Association.

BURACK, J., BARRETT, D.C., STALL, R.D., CHESNEY, M.A., EKSTRAND, M.L. and COATES, T.J. (1993) 'Depressive symptoms and CD4 lymphocyte decline among HIV-infected men', *Journal of the American Medical Association*, **270**, pp. 2568–73.

CASSEL, J. (1976) 'The contribution of the social environment to host resistance: the fourth Wade Hampton Frost Lecture', *American Journal of Epidemiology*, **104**, pp. 107–23.

COATES, T.J., McKUSICK, L., KUNO, R. and STITES, D.P. (1989) 'Stress reduction training changed number of sexual partners but not immune function in men with HIV', *American Journal of Public Health*, **79**, pp. 885–87.

COBB, S.C. (1976) 'Social support as a moderator of life stress', *Psychosomatic Medicine*, **38**, pp. 300–14.

COHEN, S. (1988) 'Psychosocial models of the role of social support in the etiology of physical disease', *Health Psychology*, **7**, pp. 269–97.

COHEN, S. and HERBERT, T.B. (1996) 'Psychological factors and physical disease from the perspective of human psychoneuroimmunology', *Annual Review of Psychology*, **47**, pp. 113–42.

DETELS, R., ENGLISH, P. and VISSCHER, B.R. (1989) 'Seroconversion, sexual activity and condom use among 2915 HIV seronegative men followed for up to 2 years', *Journal of Acquired Immune Deficiency Syndrome*, **2**, pp. 77–83.

DETELS, R., ENGLISH, P.A., GIORGO, J.V., VISSCHER, B.R., FAHEY, J.L., TAYLOR, J.M., DUDLEY, J.P., NISHANIAN, P., MUNOZ, A. and PHAIR, J.P. (1988) 'Patterns of CD4+ cell changes after HIV-1 infection indicate the existence of a co-determinant of AIDS', *Journal of Acquired Immune Deficiency Syndrome*, **1**, pp. 390–95.

EVANS, D.W., LESERMAN, J., PERKINS, D.O., STERN, R.A., MURPHY, C., TAMUL, K., LIAO, D., VAN DER HORST, C.M., HALL, C.D., FOLDS, J.D., GOLDEN, R.N. and PETITTO, J.M. (1995) 'Stress-associated reductions in cytotoxic T lymphocytes and natural killer cells in asymptomatic HIV infection', *American Journal of Psychiatry*, **152**, pp. 543–50.

FOLKMAN, S. and LAZARUS, R.S. (1980) 'An analysis of coping in a middle-aged community sample', *Journal of Health and Social Behavior*, **21**, pp. 219–39.

GARDNER, L.L., BRUNDAGE, J.F., NCNEIL, J.G. *et al.* (1992) 'Predictors of HIV-1 disease progression in early and late stage patients: the US Army natural history cohort', *Journal of Acquired Immune Deficiency Syndrome*, **5**, pp. 782–93.

GLASER, R., KIECOLT-GLASER, J.K., SPEICHER, C.E. and HOLLIDAY, J.E. (1985) 'Stress, loneliness and changes in herpes virus latency', *Journal of Behavioral Medicine*, **8**, pp. 249–60.

GLASER, R., RICE, J., SHERIDAN, J., FERTEL, R. and STOUT, J.C. (1987) 'Stress-related immune suppression: health implications', *Brain Behaviour and Immunology*, **1**, pp. 7–20.

GLASER, R., PEARSON, G.R., JONES, J.F., HILLHOUSE, J. and KENNEDY, S. (1991) 'Stress-related activation of Epstein–Barr virus', *Brain Behaviour and Immunology*, **5**, pp. 219–32.

GLASER, R., PEARSON, G.R., BONNEAU, R.H., ESTERLING, B.A., ATKINSON, C. and KIECOLT-GLASER, J.K. (1993) 'Stress and the memory T-cell response to the Epstein–Barr virus in healthy medical students', *Health Psychology*, **12**, pp. 435–42.

GOODKIN, K., FLETCHER, M.A. and COHEN, N. (1995) 'Clinical aspects of psychoneuroimmunology', *Lancet*, **345**, pp. 183–84.

GOODKIN, K., BLANEY, N.T., FEASTER, D., FLETCHER, M.A., BAUM, M.K., MANTEROATIENZA, E., KLIMAS, N.G., MILLON, C., SZAPOCZNIK, J. and EISDORFER, C. (1992) 'Active coping style is associated with natural killer cell cytotoxicity in asymptomatic HIV-1 seropositive homosexual men', *Journal of Psychosomatic Research*, **36**, pp. 635–50.

GREGORY, M.D. and SMELTZER, M.A. (1983) *Psychiatry: essentials of clinical practice*, Boston MA: Little Brown.

HERBERT, T.B. and COHEN, S. (1993) 'Depression and immunity: a meta-analytic review', *Psychological Bulletin*, **113**, pp. 472–86.

HISLOP, G.T., WAXLER, N.E., COLDMAN, A.S., ELWOOD, J.M. and KAN, L. (1987) 'The prognostic significance of psychosocial factors in women with breast cancer', *Journal of Chronic Diseases*, **40**, pp. 729–35.

HOUSE, J.S., LANDIS, K.R. and UMBERSON, D. (1988) 'Social relationships and health', *Science*, **241**, pp. 540–45.

HUNT, J.C. and WALLER, G. (1992) 'Psychological factors in recurrent uncomplicated urinary tract infection', *British Journal of Urology*, **69**, pp. 460–64.

IRONSON, G., LaPERRIERE, A., ANTONI, M., O'HEARN, P., SCHNEIDERMAN, N., KLIMAS, N. and FLETCHER, M.A. (1990) 'Changes in immune and psychological measures as a function of anticipation and reaction to news of HIV-1 antibody status', *Psychosomatic Medicine*, **52**, pp. 247–70.

IRONSON, G., FRIEDMAN, A., KLIMAS, N., ANTONI, M., FLETCHER, M.A., LaPERRIERE, A., SIMONEAU, J. and SCHNEIDERMAN, N. (1994) 'Distress, denial and low adherence to behavioural interventions predict faster disease progression in gay men infected with human immunodeficiency virus', *International Journal of Behavioural Medicine*, **1**, pp. 90–105.

KEMENY, M.E., WEINER, H., DURAN, R., TAYLOR, S.E., VISSCHER, B. and FAHEY, J.L. (1995) 'Immune system changes following the death of a partner in HIV positive gay men', *Psychosomatic Medicine*, **57**, pp. 547–54.

KIECOLT-GLASER, J.K., GARNER, W., SPEICHER, C.E., PENN, G.M., HOLLIDAY, J. and GLASER, R. (1984) 'Psychosocial modifiers of immunocompetence in medical students', *Psychosomatic Medicine*, **46**, pp. 7–14.

KIECOLT-GLASER, J.K., STRAIN, E., STOUT, J. and TARR, K. (1986) 'Modulation of cellular immunity in medical students', *Journal of Behavioral Medicine*, **9**, pp. 5–21.

LaPERRIERE, A.R., ANTONI, M.H., SCHNEIDERMAN, N., IRONSON, G., KLIMAS, N., CARALIS, P. and FLETCHER, M.A. (1990) 'Exercise intervention attenuates emotional distress and natural killer cell decrements following notification of positive serologic status for HIV-1', *Biofeedback and Self-Regulation*, **15**, pp. 229–42.

LaPERRIERE, A., FLETCHER, M.A., ANTONI, M.H., KLIMAS, N.G. and IRONSON, G. (1991) 'Aerobic exercise training in an AIDS risk group', *International Journal of Sports Medicine*, **12**, pp. s53–57.

LUTGENDORF, S.K., ANTONI, M.H., IRONSON, G., KLIMAS, N., KUMAR, M., STARR, K., McCABE, P. and CLEVEN, K. (1997) 'Cognitive-behavioural stress management decreases dysphoric mood and herpes simplex virus – type 2 antibody titers in symptomatic HIV-seropositive gay men', *Journal of Consulting and Clinical Psychology*, **65**, pp. 31–43.

LYKETSOS, C.G., HOOVER, D.R., GUCCIONE, M., SENTERFITT, W., DEW, M.A., WESCH, J., VANRADEN, M.J., TREISMAN, G.J. and MORGENSTERN, H. (1993) 'Depressive symptoms as predictors of medical outcomes in HIV infection', *Journal of the American Medical Association*, **270**, pp. 2563–67.

McKINNON, W., WEISSE, C.S., REYNOLDS, C.P., BOWLES, C.A. and BAUM, A. (1989) 'Chronic stress, leukocyte subpopulations, and humoral response to latent viruses', *Health Psychology*, **8**, pp. 389–402.

MAYNE, T.J., VITTINGHOFF, E., CHESNEY, M.A., BARRETT, D.C. and COATES, T.J. (1996) 'Depressive affect and survival among gay and bisexual men infected with HIV', *Archives of Internal Medicine*, **156**, pp. 2233–38.

MULDER, C.L., ANTONI, M.H., DUIVENVOORDEN, H.J., KAUFFMANN, R.H. and GOODKIN, K. (1995) 'Active confrontational coping predicts decreased clinical progression over a one-year period in HIV-infected homosexual men', *Journal of Psychosomatic Research*, **39**, pp. 957–65.

MUNOZ, A., CAREY, V., SAAH, A.J., PHAIR, J.P., KINSLEY, L.A., FAHEY, J.L., GINZBURG, H.M. and POLK, B.F. (1988) 'Predictors of decline in CD4 lymphocytes in a cohort of homosexual men infected with human immunodeficiency virus', *Journal of Acquired Immune Deficiency Syndrome*, **1**, pp. 396–404.

PERRY, S., FISHMAN, B., JACOBSBERG, L. and FRANCES, A. (1992) 'Relationships over 1 year between lymphocyte subsets and psychosocial variables among adults with infection by human immunodeficiency virus', *Archives of General Psychiatry*, **49**, pp. 396–401.

PHAIR, J., JACOBSON, L. and DETELS, R. (1991) 'Acquired immune deficiency symdrome occuring within 5 years of infection with human immunodeficiency virus type 1: the multicenter AIDS cohort study', *Journal of Acquired Immune Deficiency Syndrome*, **5**, pp. 490–96.

RABKIN, J.G., WILLIAMS, J.B.W., REMIEN, R.H., GOETZ, R., KERTZNER, R. and GORMAN, J.M. (1991) 'Depression, distress, lymphocyte subsets and human immunodeficiency virus symptoms on two occasions in HIV positive homosexual men', *Archives of General Psychiatry*, **48**, pp. 111–19.

REED, G.M., KEMENY, M.E., TAYLOR, S.E., WANG, H.J. and VISSCHER, B.R. (1994) 'Realistic acceptance as a predictor of decreased survival time in gay men with AIDS', *Health Psychology*, **13**, pp. 299–307.

ROTHENBURG, R., WOELFEL, M., STONEBURNER, R. *et al.* (1987) 'Survival with the acquired immunodeficiency syndrome', *New England Journal of Medicine*, **317**, pp. 1297–1302.

SAHS, J.A., GOETZ, R., REDDY, M., RABKIN, J.G., WILLIAMS, J.B.W., KERTZNER, R. and GORMAN, J.M. (1994) 'Psychological distress and natural killer cells in gay men with and without HIV infection', *American Journal of Psychiatry*, **151**, pp. 1479–84.

SEGERSTROM, S.C., TAYLOR, S.E., KEMENY, M.E., REED, G.M. and VISSCHER, B.R. (1996) 'Causal attributions predict rate of immune decline in HIV-seropositive gay men', *Health Psychology*, **15**, pp. 485–93.

SOLANO, L., COSTA, M., SALVATI, S., CODA, R., AIUTA, F., MEZZAROMA, I. and BERTINI, M. (1993) 'Psychosocial factors and clinical evolution in HIV-1 infection: a longitudinal study', *Journal of Psychosomatic Research*, **37**, pp. 39–51.

STEIN, M., MILLER, A.H. and TRESTMAN, R.L. (1991) 'Depression, the immune system and health and illness', *Archives of General Psychiatry*, **48**, pp. 171–77.

THORNTON, S., EASTERBROOK, P., TROOP, M., BURGESS, A., CATALÁN, J. and BUTTON, J. (submitted) 'Psychological variables and HIV infection: a study of their effects on disease progression among long-term infected individuals', *Psychological Medicine*.

VEDHARA, K., NOTT, K.H., BRADBEER, C.S., DAVIDSON, E.A.F., ONG, E.L.C., SNOW, M.H., PALMER, D. and NAYAGAM, A.T. (1997) 'Greater emotional distress is associated with accelerated CD4+ cell decline in HIV infection', *Journal of Psychosomatic Research*, **42**, pp. 379–90.

VERBRUGGE, L.M. (1979) 'Marital status and health', *Journal of Marriage and the Family*, **41**, pp. 267–85.

Notes on Contributors

Adrian trained as a doctor and hospital specialist. He has continued his career to this day, after being diagnosed HIV positive in 1990 (with a CD4 count of 30), and with AIDS in 1992.

José Luis Ayuso Mateos is professor of psychiatry at the University of Cantabria, Spain, and a researcher at the Clinical and Social Psychiatry Research Unit of Cantabria (the World Health Organization Collaborating Centre for Research and Training in Mental Health in Spain). His main current research areas are the study of the prevalence of neuropsychiatric disorders in patients with HIV infection and the outcome of depressive disorders in the general population.

Frans van den Boom has been interested in the psychosocial aspects of HIV infection and AIDS for many years and has published extensively on such topics as long-term planning in the field of HIV and AIDS, psychiatric and psychological disorders, death and dying, physician-assisted suicide and euthanasia. He is the director of policy, planning and organizational development for the Netherlands Red Cross.

Adrian Burgess is a clinical psychologist and senior lecturer at Imperial College, London. In his clinical capacity he has worked with people with HIV infection since 1987. His research interests include the neuropsychology and psychosocial impact of HIV infection, with a particular interest in quality-of-life issues. He has co-authored more than twenty research articles on HIV and has written a book with Drs Catalán and Klimes entitled *The Psychological Medicine of HIV Infection*.

José Catalán is a psychiatrist involved in both clinical and research work, with a predominant interest in general hospital psychiatry. He has been involved in HIV-related work since the mid-1980s, and since 1989 has worked as a liaison psychiatrist at the Chelsea and Westminster Hospital, the largest British centre for the care of people with HIV infection. Dr Catalán has published extensively on the mental health consequences of HIV infection and how to treat them. He is reader in psychiatry at Imperial College, London.

Simon Dupont is a chartered clinical psychologist who has worked in the field of HIV since 1995, having previously completed a PhD studying psychological adaptation to chronic illness. His main areas of interest also include sexual and relationship problems in HIV, schema-focused therapy and the interface in medical and psychological service provision.

Barbara Hedge has been involved in working with people with HIV infection and carrying out research into the psychological consequences of the infection since the early 1980s. She is consultant clinical psychologist and head of psychology in the department of infection and immunity at St Bartholomew's Hospital. Her current research interests include treatment adherence to antiretrovirals and its determinants, and the impact of HIV infection on relatives and carers.

Erik Hochheimer is a general practitioner who has been working in the field of HIV and AIDS for many years. As a doctor, he has often been confronted with questions about death, dying, suicide, and euthanasia. As well as his general practice work, Erik Hochheimer is affiliated to the Department of General Practice, University of Amsterdam.

George Hodson has worked as a copywriter and creative director in the United Kingdom, the United States and Asia. Since his retirement in 1989, he has done voluntary work as an AIDS activist by helping to put a face to the pandemic. He gives frequent talks to various groups and schools, and has worked with a wide range of media outlets. He is also an artist working in the medium of collage.

Carole Mitchell is a specialist registrar in psychiatry with a special interest in general hospital psychiatry. She has been involved in HIV care since 1994, initially in the United States, where she had a fellowship in liaison psychiatry in Houston, Texas, developing mental health services for women with HIV infection; and more recently at the Chelsea and Westminster Hospital in London.

Deepti Shah is a clinical psychologist with a special interest in sexual health in HIV and AIDS. She has extensive experience in research and clinical work, particularly in connection with psychological interventions for reducing the risk of HIV transmission.

Lorraine Sherr is a senior lecturer and clinical psychologist at the Royal Free Hospital School of Medicine. She is an editor of the international journal *AIDS Care* and also edits *Psychology, Health and Medicine*. Dr Sherr has conducted national and international research and policy studies, recently coordinating a European study on HIV testing in pregnancy. She is a Churchill Fellow for work on AIDS in obstetrics and paediatrics and has authored numerous texts on this subject.

Ashok N. Singh has had extensive experience in the treatment of psychiatric illness in patients with HIV and AIDS, and is currently consultant psychiatrist in South Lincolnshire Community and Mental Health Services NHS Trust. His current interests include psychopharmacology in the medically ill, cultural aspects of psychiatry and sexual dysfunction.

Fabrizio Starace is assistant director at the Regional Coordinating Centre for AIDS Policy in Naples, Italy. Additionally, as medical officer for the World Health Organization (Geneva), Fabrizio Starace has participated in the co-ordination of the WHO neuropsychiatric AIDS study. Since 1996 he has been working as an honorary lecturer at the Royal Free Hospital School of Medicine in London, researching into suicidal behaviours and end-of-life issues in HIV and AIDS.

Susan Thornton is a consultant clinical psychologist at the Psychological Medicine Unit, Chelsea and Westminster Hospital. She has worked in the HIV area since 1991, having previously worked with a wide variety of clinical groups. The clinical psychologists in the team are particularly well known for their expertise in cognitive-behavioural therapy, neuropsychology and sexual risk reduction.

Val was diagnosed HIV positive at the age of 15. She went on to nurture interests in heroin, A levels and university. Ten years on she remains largely well and has finally given up smack to devote attention to her PhD.

Edwina Williams is a specialist registrar in psychiatry with a special interest in general hospital psychiatry. She has extensive experience in the psychiatric care of HIV infection.

Index

Notes: 1. **Emboldened** page numbers indicate major treatment of topics, mainly chapters. 2. Most references are to *United Kingdom* and *gay and bisexual men*, except where otherwise specified.

Milton Keynes UK
Ingram Content Group UK Ltd.
UKHW040712141024
449569UK00012B/610